NEUROLOGY

MEDICAL EXAMINATION REVIEW

NEUROLOGY

SPECIALTY BOARD REVIEW

THIRD EDITION

600

Multiple Choice Questions With
Referenced Explanatory Answers

BARBARA S. GIESSER, M.D.
Assistant Professor of Neurology

MINDY AISEN, M.D.
Assistant Professor of Neurology

LABE C. SCHEINBERG, M.D.
Professor of Neurology and
Rehabilitation Medicine
Department of Neurology and
The Research and Training Center
Albert Einstein College of Medicine
of Yeshiva University

MEDICAL EXAMINATION PUBLISHING COMPANY

ISBN 0-8385-6692-8

Library of Congress Cataloging in Publication Data

Medical examination review: specialty board review – Flushing, N.Y.:
Medical Examination Pub. Co., 1964-<1978 >
v. <1-11 > : ill. ; 22 cm
LC holdings recorded in Shelflist only as of 3/23/82.
Earlier vols. have title: Medical examination review book : specialty board review.
Includes earlier eds. of some vols.
Later vols. published in Garden City, N.Y.
Includes biographical references.
Contents: [1] Internal medicine. <6th ed. 1978> - [2] Pediatrics. <4th ed. 1974> - [3] Obstetrics and gynecology. <5th ed. 1977> - [4] Pathology. <4th ed 1976> - [5] Surgery. <5th ed. 1973> - [6] Neurology. < 2d ed. 1972> - [7] Family practice. < 3rd ed. 1973> - [8] Dermatology. <2d ed. 1974> - [9] Psychiatry. <2d ed. 1977> - [10] cardiology. <1975> - [11] Gastroenterology. <1977>
1. Medicine – Examinations, questions, etc. I. Medical Examination Publishing Co.
RC58.M422 616'.0076 – dc19 67-1856 AACR 2 MARC

Current printing (last digit)
10 9 8 7 6 5 4 3 2 1

Manufactured in the United States of America

To our families

Contents

Preface

There are no short cuts to the process of learning! The material on the following pages is not designed to provide the reader with an opportunity to escape from learning basic information that can only be obtained from textbooks. The purpose of this text is to encourage the readers to detect areas of weakness in their understanding of subject matter so that they may return to their texts for a more comprehensive review of the subject. Crossword puzzles are not designed to teach basic English, examination review books do not teach a basic understanding of the subject. However, the following pages will provide an interesting challenge to students as well as an opportunity to improve your skills with multiple-choice examinations.

The completely referenced form of the answer material is provided to facilitate the reader in checking areas of weakness. Do not compromise by simply looking up the correct answers—the mature approach is to return to your textbook. The authors have provided you with a time-saving device in rapidly finding a source of information. While testing your memory be aware of the textbook and journal as being the ultimate source of your fund of knowledge.

The following test material will give you an opportunity to determine your ability to read, digest, and comprehend the vast accumulation of available knowledge. Don't be discouraged if you are unable to achieve a perfect test score; indeed be stimulated to learn the material by referring to your textbooks and journals. Successfully solving the problems in this text will surely give you satisfaction.

Acknowledgment

We would like to acknowledge the contribution of Dr. Alex Aisen, Assistant Professor of Radiology, University of Michigan, who provided many of the radiographic pictures used in this edition. We also thank Dr. Philip Kanof and Ms. Nancy Denner for their assistance in preparing this manuscript.

1 NEUROANATOMY

DIRECTIONS: Each of the questions or incomplete statements below is followed by a list of suggested answers or completions. Select the **one** that is best in each case.

---

1. Internal arcuate fibers decussate in the medulla and form the
   A. medial lemniscus
   B. medial longitudinal fasciculus
   C. arcuate nucleus
   D. vestibulospinal tract
   E. none of the above

2. The auditory pathway passes through all of the structures listed below EXCEPT
   A. medial lemniscus
   B. lateral lemniscus
   C. lateral geniculate body
   D. trapezoid body
   E. none of the above

3. The cerebellar lesion that would be expected to produce the most extensive disorders of eye movement would be in the
   - **A.** nodulus
   - **B.** flocculus
   - **C.** vermis
   - **D.** emboliform nucleus
   - **E.** none of the above

4. The lenticulo striate arteries
   - **A.** supply the anterior part of the anterior limb of the internal capsule
   - **B.** supply the posterior part of the posterior limb of the internal capsule
   - **C.** supply the anterior part of the posterior limb of the internal capsule
   - **D.** arise from the posterior cerebral arteries
   - **E.** none of the above

5. Descending fibers of the substantia gelatinosa become the
   - **A.** inferior vestibular nucleus
   - **B.** medial vestibular nucleus
   - **C.** spinal trigeminal nucleus
   - **D.** nucleus ambiguus
   - **E.** none of the above

6. The substantia gelatinosa receives primarily the fibers of the
   - **A.** lateral spinothalamic tract
   - **B.** dorsal roots mediating pain and temperature
   - **C.** nucleus of Clarke
   - **D.** anterior spinothalamic tract
   - **E.** none of the above

7. Underlying the ala cinerea lies the
   - **A.** hypoglossal nucleus
   - **B.** dorsal efferent nucleus of the vagus
   - **C.** nucleus ambiguous
   - **D.** area postrema
   - **E.** none of the above

8. The H_2 bundle of Forel is also known as the
   A. lenticular fasciculus
   B. ansa lenticularis
   C. thalamic fasciculus
   D. subthalamic fasciculus
   E. none of the above

9. To which does the inferior colliculus project?
   A. Lateral lemniscus
   B. Medial geniculate
   C. Lateral geniculate
   D. Medial lemniscus
   E. None of the above

10. The anterior limb of the internal capsule does not carry
    A. thalamic radiations
    B. frontopontine fibers
    C. corticobulbar fibers
    D. fibers from the orbital cortex
    E. none of the above

11. The lateral lemniscus projects to the
    A. lateral geniculate nucleus of the thalamus
    B. medial geniculate nucleus of the thalamus
    C. VPL nucleus of the thalamus
    D. VPM nucleus of the thalamus
    E. VL nucleus of the thalamus

12. Pain, temperature and touch sensation from the face project to
    A. VPL nucleus of the thalamus
    B. VPM nucleus of the thalamus
    C. VL nucleus of the thalamus
    D. VA nucleus of the thalamus
    E. none of the above

13. The fornicate lobe
    A. contains the cingulate, isthmus, and hippocampal gyri
    B. is part of the frontal lobe
    C. is part of the cerebellar vermis
    D. is part of the occipital lobe
    E. none of the above

14. The average weight of the American male brain is
A. 1100 gm
B. 1300 gm
C. 1500 gm
D. 1800 gm
E. none of the above

15. The dentate nucleus of the cerebellum projects mainly to the red nucleus and the
A. globus pallidus
B. VL nucleus of the thalamus
C. vestibular nuclei
D. VA nucleus of the thalamus
E. none of the above

16. The median forebrain bundle arises in the
A. medial olfactory area
B. lateral olfactory area
C. anterior thalamus
D. hippocampus
E. none of the above

17. The cell type which is a sine qua non for cortex is the
A. pyramidal cell
B. stellate cell
C. horizontal cells of Cajal
D. spindle cells
E. none of the above

18. Lissauer's tract
A. receives fibers from the substantia gelatinosa
B. sends fibers to the substantia gelatinosa
C. receives fibers from the nucleus proprius
D. contains only myelinated fibers
E. none of the above

19. The recurrent artery of Heubner
A. arises from the internal carotid artery
B. arises from the anterior communicating artery
C. arises from the anterior choroidal artery
D. arises from the anterior cerebral artery
E. none of the above

20. Visual cortex
    A. is thicker than average cortex
    B. is thinner than average cortex
    C. is the same thickness as average cortex
    D. occupies 40% of the entire cortex
    E. occupies 20% of the entire cortex

21. The cerebellum receives inputs from each of the following sources through the inferior peduncle EXCEPT
    A. the dorsal spinocerebellar tract
    B. the ventral spinocerebellar tract
    C. the inferior olive
    D. the cuneocerebellar tract
    E. none of the above

22. The frontal lobe contains what percent of the total surface area of the cortex?
    A. 20%
    B. 40%
    C. 50%
    D. 60%
    E. None of the above

23. Parallel fibers of the cerebellum are axons of
    A. basket cells
    B. granule cells
    C. stellate cells
    D. Purkinje cells
    E. none of the above

24. Adrenergic fibers include the
    A. preganglionic sympathetics
    B. preganglionic parasympathetics
    C. postganglionic parasympathetics
    D. postganglionic sympathetics
    E. none of the above

25. The spinotectal tract
    A. terminates in the inferior colliculus
    B. originates in the nucleus proprius
    C. lies lateral to the lateral spinothalamic tract
    D. projects to the superior colliculus
    E. none of the above

26. The cell bodies of optic nerve fibers are the
  - **A.** rods and cones of the retina
  - **B.** bipolar cells of the retina
  - **C.** ganglion cells of the retina
  - **D.** horizontal cells of the retina
  - **E.** none of the above

27. Which of the following is the most medial cerebellar nucleus?
  - **A.** Emboliform nucleus
  - **B.** Fastigial nucleus
  - **C.** Dentate nucleus
  - **D.** Globose nucleus

28. The efferent neurones of the cerebellar cortex are the
  - **A.** Purkinje cells
  - **B.** climbing fibers
  - **C.** mossy fibers
  - **D.** Golgi cells
  - **E.** none of the above

29. The "artery of internal hemorrhage" or "artery of Charcot" is a branch of
  - **A.** the lenticulostriate group
  - **B.** the anterior chorioidal artery
  - **C.** the thalamogeniculate group
  - **D.** the anteromedial group
  - **E.** none of the above

30. The genu of the internal capsule carries
  - **A.** anterior thalamic radiations
  - **B.** frontopontine fibers
  - **C.** corticobulbar fibers
  - **D.** corticorubral fibers
  - **E.** none of the above

31. Inferior retinal fibers (superior visual fields) are projected to
  - **A.** inferior calcarine cortex
  - **B.** superior calcarine cortex
  - **C.** anterior calcarine cortex
  - **D.** posterior calcarine cortex
  - **E.** none of the above

DIRECTIONS: For each of the questions or incomplete statements below, **one or more** of the answers or completions given is correct. Select

(A) if only 1, 2, and 3 are correct
(B) if only 1 and 3 are correct
(C) if only 2 and 4 are correct
(D) if only 4 is correct
(E) if all are correct

32. The blood-brain barrier

1. is absent at the supraoptic crest
2. is composed, in part, of arachnoid membrane
3. stains after systemic injection of trypan blue
4. is more permeable to acidic (negatively charged) dyes

33. Fibers of the cuneocerebellar tract

1. arise from cells in the dorsal nucleus of Clarke
2. are the upper limb equivalent of the anterior spinocerebellar tract
3. convey information from Golgi tendon organs
4. enter the cerebellum via the inferior cerebellar peduncle

34. The inferior cerebellar peduncle

1. is also known as the brachium pontis
2. contains primarily fibers from the anterior spinocerebellar tract
3. is the major connection between the cerebellum and the pons
4. is the pathway through which the posterior spinocerebellar tract enters the cerebellum

35. The dentate nucleus

1. is the site of the major efferent pathway for the cerebellum
2. sends most of its fibers out through the brachium conjunctivum
3. is lateral to the emboliform nucleus
4. projects primarily to the ventral anterior nucleus of the thalamus

---

DIRECTIONS: Each group of questions below consists of a list of lettered headings followed by a list of numbered words or statements. For **each** numbered word or statement, select the **one** lettered heading that is most closely associated with it. Each lettered heading may be selected once, more than once, or not at all.

Match the cerebral structure with the source of its major blood supply.

A. Internal carotid artery
B. Middle cerebral artery
C. Posterior cerebral artery
D. Anterior cerebral artery

36. Anterior limb of internal capsule
37. Thalamus
38. Globus pallidus
39. Hypothalamus

Match the peripheral receptor with the statement that best applies to it.

A. Largest encapsulated receptor
B. Group 1a fibers
C. Two-point discrimination
D. Free nerve ending
E. Group 1b fibers

40. Meissner's corpuscle
41. Pacinian corpuscle
42. Tactile disc of Merkel
43. Annulospiral afferents
44. Golgi tendon organ

Match the cell type with the corresponding lamina of Rexed.

A. Lamina VII
B. Lamina II
C. Lamina IX
D. Lamina IV
E. Lamina V

45. Substantia gelatinosa
46. Alpha motor neurons
47. Renshaw cells
48. Nucleus proprius

Match the site of the lesion with the clinical effects.

A. Lateral lemniscus
B. Spiral ganglion
C. Dorsal cochlear nucleus
D. Temporal lobe

49. Ipsilateral deafness
50. Contralateral deafness (partial)
51. Contralateral deficit in sound localization

Match the anatomic site with its function.

A. Feeding center
B. Satiety center
C. ADH secretion
D. Heat dissipation
E. Oxytocin secretion

52. Ventromedial hypothalamic nucleus
53. Supraoptic nucleus
54. Lateral hypothalamic nucleus
55. Paraventricular nucleus

Match the site of the lesion with the clinical picture.

A. Adie's pupil
B. Horner's pupil
C. Argyll-Robertson pupil
D. Marcus-Gunn pupil

56. Dorsal midbrain
57. Superior cervical ganglion
58. Postganglionic short ciliary nerves

Match each function with its cortical area.

A. 39, 40
B. 18, 19
C. 4
D. 3, 2, 1
E. 6, 8
F. 17
G. 41, 42

59. Somesthetic cortex
60. Speech association
61. Conscious vision
62. Visual association
63. Auditory cortex
64. Primary motor
65. Supplementary motor

Match each thalamic nucleus with the cortical area to which it projects.

A. 41, 42
B. 17
C. 3, 2, 1
D. 4, 6, 8
E. 39, 40

66. Posteromedial ventral nucleus
67. Posterolateral ventral nucleus
68. Medial geniculate
69. Lateral geniculate
70. Anterior and lateral ventral nuclei

A. Inferior cerebellar peduncle
B. Middle cerebellar peduncle
C. Superior cerebellar peduncle

71. Pontocerebellar fibers
72. Dorsal spinocerebellar tract
73. Arcuatocerebellar fibers
74. Cerebellotectal fibers
75. Cerebellotegmental fibers
76. Olivocerebellar fibers
77. Dentatorubral fibers
78. Dorsal superficial arcuate fibers
79. Ventral superficial arcuate fibers
80. Dentatothalamic fibers
81. Ventral spinocerebellar

DIRECTIONS: Each set of lettered headings below is followed by a list of numbered words or phrases. For **each** numbered word or phrase select

(A) if the item is associated with A **only**
(B) if the item is associated with B **only**
(C) if the item is associated with **both** A and B
(D) if the item is associated with **neither** A nor B

A. Visual system
B. Auditory system
C. Both
D. Neither

82. Medial geniculate
83. Inferior colliculus
84. Lateral geniculate
85. Medial longitudinal fasciculus

2 NEUROPATHOLOGY

DIRECTIONS: Each of the questions or incomplete statements below is followed by a list of suggested answers or completions. Select the **one** that is best in each case.

---

86. Bunina bodies are found in
- **A.** Huntington's disease
- **B.** Pelizaeus-Merzbacher disease
- **C.** amyotrophic lateral sclerosis
- **D.** Jakob-Creutzfeld disease
- **E.** Wilson's disease

87. Sea-blue histiocytes are found in
- **A.** Tay-Sach's disease
- **B.** Niemann-Pick disease
- **C.** metachromatic leukodystrophy
- **D.** Krabbe's disease
- **E.** Hurler's disease

88. Marek's disease of turkeys may serve as an animal model for
- **A.** multiple sclerosis
- **B.** Binswanger's disease
- **C.** Guillain-Barré syndrome
- **D.** Marchiafava-Bignami disease
- **E.** diabetic neuropathy

89. The clinical syndrome of constricted visual fields, paresthesias, and cerebellar ataxia (Hunter-Russel syndrome) is caused by toxicity with

A. lead
B. methylmercury
C. phosphorus
D. thallium
E. arsenic

90. Retinitis pigmentosa, acanthocytosis, and spinocerebellar signs are most characteristic of

A. ceroid lipofuscinosis
B. Wolman's disease
C. Bassen-Kornzweig
D. Tangier disease
E. Kearns-Sayre syndrome

91. Which of the following is a false statement about vertebrate vision?

A. Rod cells are more numerous than cone cells
B. Dopamine has been identified as a retinal neurotransmitter
C. "Visual excitation" by light inhibits the release of chemical transmitter
D. Cone cells are receptors for photopic vision
E. None of the above

92. Polar spongioblastomas

A. arise in the first or second decade and are usually located in the region of the third or fourth ventricle
B. have a mode of spread which resembles the medulloblastoma
C. characteristically contain giant or multinucleated cells
D. A and B
E. B and C

93. Oligodendroglioma
A. usually presents as a well-defined, circumscribed mass which is often cystic. Microscopically, perinuclear halos are characteristic
B. frequently contains foci of hemorrhage and calcification
C. is significantly more common in childhood
D. A and B
E. B and C

94. The subependymal giant cell astrocytoma
A. characteristically is associated with tuberous sclerosis
B. characteristically is associated with neurofibromatosis
C. frequently exhibits malignant changes (necrosis, cellular anaplasia)
D. is not associated with hydrocephalus
E. none of the above

95. Which of the following is more common in females?
A. Medulloblastoma
B. Glioblastoma
C. Intraspinal astrocytoma
D. Intracranial schwannoma
E. A and D

96. Segmental demyelination is an outstanding characteristic of all but one of the following neuropathies
A. Guillain-Barré syndrome
B. thiamine deficiency
C. diphtheria
D. metachromatic leukodystrophy

97. Hallervorden-Spatz disease
A. has iron deposits in the basal ganglia
B. has status spongiosus of the cortex
C. has peripheral chromatolysis of the anterior horn cells
D. is seen in senile patients
E. none of the above

98. Nissl granules are usually not found in which of these locations?
   - A. Cytoplasm
   - B. Cortical neurons
   - C. Axon hillock
   - D. Dendrite
   - E. Any of the above

99. The central nervous system lesions in toxoplasmosis
   - A. often calcify
   - B. consist of both large and miliary granulomata
   - C. are accompanied by diffuse meningeal infiltration
   - D. none of the above
   - E. all of the above

100. Extrapyramidal syndromes may be seen following which of the following intoxications?
   - A. Carbon monoxide
   - B. Methyl alcohol
   - C. Ethyl alcohol
   - D. Magnesium
   - E. None of the above

101. Which of the following is not seen after severe anoxia?
   - A. Purkinje cell loss
   - B. Laminar necrosis
   - C. Chromatolysis in anterior horn cells
   - D. Cell loss in Ammon's horn
   - E. Cell loss in the globus pallidus

102. Which one of the following is not seen in lathyrism?
   - A. Optic atrophy
   - B. Spinocerebellar tract degeneration
   - C. Lateral cortical spinal tract degeneration
   - D. Posterior column degeneration
   - E. None of the above

103. Which of the following is not usually found in subacute combined degeneration of the nervous system?
   - A. Wallerian degeneration in the dorsal cord
   - B. Normal meninges
   - C. Degeneration of the medullary pyramids
   - D. Sparing of the spinothalamic tract
   - E. None of the above

104. The myelin-forming cell of the central nervous system is believed to be the
- **A.** oligodendroglial cell
- **B.** protoplasmic astrocyte
- **C.** microglial cell
- **D.** Schwann cell
- **E.** none of the above

105. Alzheimer type II glia are found in which one of the following?
- **A.** Kraepelin's disease
- **B.** Metachromatic leukodystrophy
- **C.** Wilson's disease
- **D.** Alzheimer's disease
- **E.** Pick's disease

106. Incisural sclerosis has been implicated as an etiologic agent in which one of the following?
- **A.** Petit-mal epilepsy
- **B.** Minimata's disease
- **C.** Psychomotor seizures
- **D.** Kuru
- **E.** Febrile seizures

107. Lewy bodies are usually found in which of the following?
- **A.** Kuru
- **B.** Devic's disease
- **C.** The substantia nigra
- **E.** None of the above

108. Following section of a peripheral nerve which of the following events occurs first?
- **A.** Disappearance of neurofibrils
- **B.** Peripheral chromatolysis
- **C.** Myelin sheath breaks down into globules
- **D.** Wallerian degeneration
- **E.** None of the above

109. The gitter cell
- **A.** usually appears within 8 hr following an infarct
- **B.** is due to central chromatolysis
- **C.** is a transformed granulocyte
- **D.** is derived from astrocytes
- **E.** none of the above

110. The effects of vascular disease on brain tissue are seen
- **A.** rarely
- **B.** in 100% of all autopsied brains
- **C.** in 25% of all autopsied brains
- **D.** only when there has been a hemiplegia
- **E.** none of the above

111. In purulent meningitis
- **A.** occlusion of subarachnoid arteries is common
- **B.** the cortex is usually only slightly involved
- **C.** the cortex is usually massively involved
- **D.** both A and B are correct
- **E.** none of the above

112. Following destruction of myelin and neurones macrophages appear
- **A.** first in the perivascular tissues
- **B.** last in the perivascular tissues
- **C.** first in the area of damage
- **D.** first in the CSF
- **E.** none of the above

113. The predominant macrophage 48 hr following an intracerebral hematoma is
- **A.** the monocyte of the bloodstream
- **B.** ependymal cell
- **C.** protoplasmic astrocyte
- **D.** fibrous astrocyte
- **E.** none of the above

114. All of the following are useful myelin stains, EXCEPT for
- **A.** Weigert
- **B.** Marchi
- **C.** PTAH
- **D.** Sudan IV
- **E.** none of the above

115. The notochord is formed in which period of development of the embryo?
- **A.** 3rd week
- **B.** 2nd month
- **C.** 3rd month
- **D.** 6th month
- **E.** 1st week

116. Radioactive albumin injected into the blood stream will equilibrate with subdural fluid within
   A. hours
   B. three days
   C. one week
   D. never
   E. none of the above

117. Posttraumatic epilepsy
   A. is rare following automobile accidents
   B. usually develops within one week of the injury
   C. usually develops 6–15 months after injury
   D. usually develops 2 years after injury
   E. none of the above

118. In Wilson's disease
   A. the ceruloplasmin is high
   B. there is cavitation in the lenticular nuclei
   C. spongy necrosis of the cortex is common
   D. Alzheimer's type I glia are common
   E. none of the above

119. Subacute sclerosing panencephalitis
   A. usually exclusively involves the posterior fossa
   B. involves the white matter with extensive areas of necrosis
   C. shows no inclusion bodies
   D. is related to mumps infection
   E. none of the above

120. Globoid bodies are characteristic of
   A. poliomyelitis
   B. Krabbe's disease
   C. Tay–Sachs disease
   D. Hallervorden–Spatz disease
   E. none of the above

121. The most common glioma is
   A. spongioblastoma polare
   B. ependymoma
   C. glioblastoma multiforme
   D. astrocytoma, grade I
   E. none of the above

122. Type A inclusion bodies are usually not seen in
   A. polio
   B. rabies
   C. herpes simplex
   D. SSPE
   E. none of the above

123. Hemangiomas
   A. are true neoplasms
   B. are developmental anomalies
   C. do not enlarge with body growth
   D. never involve the spinal cord
   E. none of the above

DIRECTIONS: For each of the questions or incomplete statements below, **one or more** of the answers or completions given is correct. Select
   (A) if only 1, 2, and 3 are correct
   (B) if only 1 and 3 are correct
   (C) if only 2 and 4 are correct
   (D) if only 4 is correct
   (E) if all are correct

---

124. Neurofibrillary tangles are present in
   1. normal aging
   2. postencephalitic Parkinson's disease
   3. Down's syndrome
   4. Alzheimer's disease

125. Hirano bodies
   1. are pathognomonic for Pick's disease
   2. are found in Jakob-Creutzfeld disease
   3. are basophilic
   4. have a highly organized crystalline fine structure

126. The spectrum of ceroid lipofuscinosis includes these syndromes
   1. Haltia-Santavori
   2. Spielmeyer-Batten-Vogt
   3. Kuf's disease
   4. Wolman's disease

Directions Summarized

(A) 1, 2, 3 only; **(B)** 1, 3 only; **(C)** 2, 4 only; **(D)** 4 only; **(E)** all

127. Aluminum
1. is present in abnormally high concentrations in the CSF of patients with Alzheimer's disease
2. has been shown to be the cause of plaques and tangles in the brains of patients with Alzheimer's disease
3. has definitely been found to be higher in the brains of patients with Alzheimer's disease than in aged matched controls
4. has been found in neurons containing neurofibrillary tangles

128. Benign intracranial hypertension
1. occurs in vitamin A toxicity
2. occurs primarily in women
3. may be associated with endocrine abnormalities
4. occurs in vitamin A deficiency

129. Characteristics of Kearns–Sayre syndrome include
1. short stature
2. mental retardation
3. deafness
4. ophthalmoplegia

130. The median eminence
1. lacks the blood–brain barrier
2. lacks neuronal cell bodies
3. is the site of hormone–releasing factors
4. is derived from the hypothalamus

DIRECTIONS: Each group of questions below consists of a list of lettered headings followed by a list of numbered words or statements. For **each** numbered word or statement, select the **one** lettered heading that is most closely associated with it. Each lettered heading may be selected once, more than once, or not at all.

A. Duchenne's
B. Myotonic dystrophy
C. Limb-girdle dystrophy
D. Nemaline myopathy

131. High arched palate and prognathia
132. Very prone to develop contractures
133. Autosomal recessive
134. Frontal balding

A. Capillary telangiectasias
B. Cavernous angiomas
C. Capillary hemangioblastoma
D. A and B

135. Von Hippel Lindau disease
136. Most common site is the pons
137. Associated rarely with Osler-Weber-Rendu syndrome
138. Histologically, vascular channels are separated by normal neural tissue
139. Often clinically silent, discovered at autopsy
140. Calcification and adjacent fibrillary gliosis
141. Associated with erythrocythemia
142. Associated with renal cell carcinoma, pancreatic cysts, retinal lesions

A. Medulloblastoma
B. Ependymoma
C. Meningioma
D. Glioblastoma
E. Schwannoma

143. Contain blepharoplasts
144. Most common intracranial brain tumor in adults
145. Most common intramedullary spinal cord tumor
146. Associated with hydrocephalus in the elderly
147. Arises in the cerebellum
148. Leptomeningeal spread is common, as is metastasis through CSF pathways
149. Contains psammoma bodies
150. Bone marrow metastasis
151. Most common primary spinal tumor

A. Cerebral amebiasis
B. Toxoplasma gondii
C. Cysticercosis
D. Echinococcus granulosus
E. None of the above

152. Nervous system lesions: small hemorrhages, meningoencephalitis, polyneuropathy
153. Systemic: perorbital edema, myalgia, eosinophilia
154. Associated with AIDS
155. Associated with eating raw pork
156. Hosts are dog and sheep; produces large cystic lesions in brain
157. Associated with lymphadenopathy and ocular lesions
158. Solitary or multiple brain abscesses in the setting of dysentery and suppurative hepatitis
159. Taenia saginata
160. Treatment with Praziquantel may be effective

A. Sphingomyelin
B. Cerebroside
C. Sulfatide
D. Glucocerebroside
E. Ganglioside
F. Zebra bodies

161. Hurler's disease
162. Niemann-Pick
163. Gaucher's disease
164. Tay-Sachs disease
165. Metachromatic leukodystrophy
166. Krabbe's leukodystrophy

Match the following diseases with their histological findings.

A. Lafora body
B. Psamomma body
C. Antoni Type A
D. Opalski cell
E. Rosenthal fibers
F. Pseudorosette formation
G. Type A inclusion body
H. Neurofibrillary tangle
I. Lewy body

167. Meningioma
168. Alzheimer's disease
169. Unverricht's myoclonus
170. Acoustic neurinoma
171. Parkinson's disease
172. Herpes simplex encephalitis
173. Piloid astrocytoma
174. Wilson's disease
175. Ependymoma

3 NEUROPHARMACOLOGY

DIRECTIONS: Each of the questions or incomplete statements below is followed by a list of suggested answers or completions. Select the **one** that is best in each case.

176. Amantadine may be classified as a
- **A.** dopamine receptor agonist
- **B.** dopamine receptor blocker
- **C.** muscarinic receptor blocker
- **D.** dopamine releaser
- **E.** none of the above

177. Bromocriptine
- **A.** unlike lisuride, is an ergot derivative which acts directly on dopamine receptors
- **B.** decreases growth-hormone levels in acromegaly
- **C.** increases the incidence of the on-off phenomenon in parkinsonism
- **D.** A and B
- **E.** none of the above

178. Phenytoin blood levels may increase
- **A.** when given concurrently with a barbiturate
- **B.** when given concurrently with chloramphenicol
- **C.** when hepatic drug metabolizing enzyme are induced by carbamezipine
- **D.** A and B

179. Valproic acid

A. reduces the metabolism of GABA
B. generally depresses serum phenobarbital levels
C. should be used exclusively for absence seizures due to the high incidence of hepatic toxicity
D. frequently produces sedation and ataxia
E. none of the above

180. In a pregnant patient with a seizure disorder treated with phenytoin

A. phenytoin should be immediately discontinued due to the associated increased incidence of birth deformities, such as cleft lip and cleft palate
B. phenytoin dosage may need to be increased due to decreased absorption during the third trimester
C. toxic effects, such as nystagmus, ataxia, hepatitis, and gingival hyperplasia, are likely to become manifest
D. phenytoin dosage should be decreased, due to increased absorption
E. none of the above

181. Hypocalcemia and osteomalacia

A. may be seen as a result of therapy with ethosuximide
B. may occur in patients receiving phenobarbital therapy
C. result from low vitamin D levels complicating phenytoin therapy
D. A and B
E. B and C

182. Pergolide

A. is a dopamine antagonist
B. reduces the severity of on-off fluctuations in Parkinson's disease
C. is a short-acting postsynaptic dopamine agonist
D. is contraindicated for patients receiving L-Dopa
E. none of the above

183. The neuroleptic malignant syndrome
- **A.** occurs in the setting of phenothiazine withdrawal
- **B.** can be exacerbated by concurrent administration of dopamine agonists, such as bromocriptine
- **C.** is characterized by severe extrapyramidal dysfunction and hyperthermia
- **D.** is a dose-related phenomenon
- **E.** none of the above

184. The side effects of bromocriptine include
- **A.** orthostatic hypotension
- **B.** nausea and vomiting
- **C.** digital vasospasm
- **D.** A and B
- **E.** A and B and C

185. The following may produce optic atrophy.
- **A.** Quinidine
- **B.** Ethanol
- **C.** Ethambutol
- **D.** A and C
- **E.** None of the above

186. Isoniazid in a dose of 6 mg/kg/day
- **A.** may produce peripheral neuropathy in 17% of patients
- **B.** produces a neuropathy characterized primarily by axonal degeneration
- **C.** lowers CNS GABA levels
- **D.** A and B
- **E.** none of the above

187. Tardive dyskinesia which persists after withdrawal of neuroleptic medication
- **A.** is best treated with anticholinergic agents
- **B.** is best treated with neuroleptic agents
- **C.** is best treated with dopaminergic agents
- **D.** never remits spontaneously
- **E.** none of the above

188. Bromocriptine
- **A.** may produce confusion and hallucinations
- **B.** should not be given in excess of 50 mg per day
- **C.** may exacerbate the disability produced by the on-off phenomenon
- **D.** does not produce ventricular ectopy, although frequently produces atrial arrhythmias
- **E.** A and D

189. Propranolol when used for the prophylaxis of migraine
- **A.** should be discontinued after 4–6 weeks of therapy if relief has not been obtained by this time
- **B.** should be discontinued after 1 year if control has been achieved, as relapse is rare
- **C.** should be used for at least 6 months, as success may progressively increase during the first year
- **D.** should not be used in excess of 160 mg/day, in order to avoid side effects such as hypotension, depression, and congestive heart failure
- **E.** none of the above

190. Which of the following would not be used in diagnosis of myasthenia gravis?
- **A.** Neostigmine
- **B.** Edrophonium
- **C.** D-tubocurarine
- **D.** Succinylcholine
- **E.** Quinine

191. Atropine is most effective as a blocking agent at
- **A.** autonomic ganglia
- **B.** adrenal medulla
- **C.** the neuromuscular junction
- **D.** the parasympathetic neuroeffector junction
- **E.** none of the above

192. Which of the following is not a catecholamine?
- **A.** Epinephrine
- **B.** Ephedrine
- **C.** Isoproterenol
- **D.** Norepinephrine
- **E.** None of the above

193. Opiates in single therapeutic doses
- **A.** do not affect the EEG
- **B.** slow the frequency and increase the amplitude of the EEG
- **C.** slow the frequency and decrease the amplitude of the EEG
- **D.** raise the frequency and increase the amplitude of the EEG
- **E.** none of the above

194. An antimuscarinic drug with CNS actions is
- **A.** atropine methylnitrate
- **B.** scopolamine
- **C.** D-Tubocurarine
- **D.** hexamethonium
- **E.** physostigmine

195. Hypertensive crisis in a patient under treatment with MAO inhibitors would most likely occur following ingestion of
- **A.** apples
- **B.** cheddar cheese
- **C.** walnuts
- **D.** smoked salmon
- **E.** white wine

196. The active substance in the food in the preceding question is
- **A.** tyramine
- **B.** 5-HT
- **C.** histamine
- **D.** tyrosine
- **E.** tryptophan

197. The efferent parasympathetic fibers may be separated into
- **A.** the cranial and lumbar outflows
- **B.** the cranial and sacral outflows
- **C.** the cervical and lumbar outflows
- **D.** the cervical and sacral outflows
- **E.** the cranial and thoracic outflows

198. The primary action of atropine at the parasympathetic neuroeffector junction is most similar to that of _____ at the neuromuscular junction.
A. D-tubocurarine
B. succinylcholine
C. decamethonium
D. hexamethonium
E. none of the above

199. The transmitter at the synapse of the motor neuron recurrent collateral and the Renshaw cell is believed to be
A. GABA
B. 5-HT
C. norepinephrine
D. glycine
E. acetylcholine

200. The primary action of hemicholinium is
A. promotion of ACh release
B. interference with ACh synthesis
C. stimulation of ACh receptors at ganglia
D. stimulation of ACh receptors at the neuromuscular junction
E. blockage of ACh receptors

201. The transmitter at parasympathetic postganglionic neuroeffector snapses is believed to be
A. muscarine
B. norepinephrine
C. epinephrine
D. acetylcholine
E. buterylcholine

202. Which of the drugs listed below does not act primarily presynaptically?
A. Guanethidine
B. Botulinus toxin
C. Reserpine
D. Pilocarpine
E. Tyramine

203. Nausea and vomiting produced by morphine are due to
- **A.** direct effects on the smooth musculature of the esophagus and stomach
- **B.** depression of hypothalamic function
- **C.** direct stimulation of the chemoreceptor trigger zone (CTZ)
- **D.** stimulation of chemoreceptive sites on the membranes of smooth muscle
- **E.** none of the above

204. All of the following drugs have parasympathomimetic actions EXCEPT
- **A.** physostigmine
- **B.** pilocarpine
- **C.** acetylcholine
- **D.** methacholine
- **E.** hemicholinium

205. Which of the following is not an intermediary in the synthesis of norepinephrine?
- **A.** Tyrosine
- **B.** Epinephrine
- **C.** Dopamine
- **D.** Dopa
- **E.** None of the above

206. The enzyme which converts 5-hydroxytryptophan (5-HTP) to 5-hydroxy-tryptamine (5-HT) is identical to the one which converts
- **A.** phenylalanine to tyrosine
- **B.** tyrosine to dopa
- **C.** dopa to dopamine
- **D.** dopamine to norepinephrine
- **E.** norepinephrine to epinephrine

207. The rate limiting step in the synthesis of norepinephrine is
- **A.** phenylalanine to tyrosine
- **B.** tyrosine to dopa
- **C.** dopa to dopamine
- **D.** dopamine to norepinephrine
- **E.** none of the above

208. Choose the wrong answer: Among the useful side effects of various antihistamines is
- **A.** suppression of motion sickness
- **B.** relief of certain parkinsonism smptoms
- **C.** symptomatic relief of tertiary syphilis
- **D.** local anesthetic activity
- **E.** none of the above

209. In humans, the enzyme chiefly responsible for the metabolism of 5-HT is
- **A.** monamine oxidase (MAO)
- **B.** catechol-o-methyltransferase
- **C.** pseudocholinesterase
- **D.** tryptophan 5-hydroxylase
- **E.** amino acid decarboxylase

210. The relatively brief duration of paralysis following a single dose of D-tubocurarine is probably due chiefly to
- **A.** renal excretion
- **B.** hydrolysis by acetylcholinesterase
- **C.** hydrolysis by pseudocholinesterase
- **D.** redistribution of drug
- **E.** hepatic metabolism

211. Zarontin is used to treat what type(s) of epilepsy(ies)?
- **A.** Grand mal
- **B.** Grand mal and petit mal
- **C.** Petit mal
- **D.** Petit mal and psychomotor
- **E.** Psychomotor

212. Whereas the transmitter at parasympathetic ganglia is acetylcholine, the transmitter at sympathetic ganglia is believed to be
- **A.** norepinephrine
- **B.** epinephrine
- **C.** muscarine
- **D.** nicotine
- **E.** acetylcholine

213. Which of the following cholinesterase inhibitors is not an organophosphorus compound?
A. Diisopropylphosphorofluoridate
B. Parathion
C. Tabun
D. Edrophonium (Tensilon)
E. Paraoxon

214. The effect of quinine in a myasthenic patient would be most similar to the effect of
A. edrophonium (Tensilon)
B. hexamethonium
C. neostigmine
D. atropine
E. D-tubocurarine

215. All of the following drugs are known to precipitate attacks of acute intermittent porphyria EXCEPT
A. phenobarbital
B. imipramine
C. diphenylhydantoin
D. guanethidine
E. glutethimide

DIRECTIONS: Match the drug from the list below which best fits the statement. Use **each** drug only once.

A. Acetylcholine
B. Norepinephrine
C. Epinephrine
D. Dopamine

216. A precursor of epinephrine
217. Synthesized by spinal motor-neurones
218. Major amine released by adrenal medullary chromaffin cells
219. Major amine released by postganglionic sympathetic neurons

DIRECTIONS: Each group of questions below consists of a list of lettered headings followed by a list of numbered words or statements. For each numbered word or statement, select the **one** lettered heading that is most closely associated with it. Each lettered heading may be selected once, more than once, or not at all.

A. Paroxysmal hemicrania
B. Chronic cluster headache
C. Acute cluster headache
D. All of the above
E. None of the above

220. Responds to treatment with indomethacin
221. Lithium is an effective treatment
222. Prednisone is an effective treatment

DIRECTIONS: For each of the questions or incomplete statements below, **one or more** of the answers or completions given is correct. Select

(A) if only 1, 2, and 3 are correct
(B) if only 1 and 3 are correct
(C) if only 2 and 4 are correct
(D) if only 4 is correct
(E) if all are correct

223. Which of these drugs may increase or precipitate vascular headache?

1. Lithium
2. Reserpine
3. Nitroglycerin
4. Inderal

224. REM latency

1. can be reduced by administration of serotonin synthesis inhibitors
2. can be reduced by administration of muscarinic receptor agonists
3. can be reduced by administration of tricyclic antidepressant drugs
4. is decreased in major depressive disorders

Directions Summarized

(A) 1, 2, 3 only; **(B)** 1, 3 only; **(C)** 2, 4 only; **(D)** 4 only; **(E)** all

225. Symptoms of opiate withdrawal include
1. seizures
2. mydriasis
3. dry skin
4. anxiety

226. Intracerebral injection of prostaglandin E
1. produces fever that is dose dependent
2. produces sedation
3. produces fever that does not respond to aspirin
4. potentiates the effects of barbiturates

227. Mediated transport across the blood-brain barrier exists for these substances
1. glucose
2. GABA
3. choline
4. glycine

228. Adenylate cyclase activity in brain has been shown to be regulated by which neurotransmitters?
1. Dopamine
2. Histamine
3. Serotonin
4. Substance P

229. Neurologic complications of fluorosis include
1. myelopathy
2. cranial nerve palsies
3. radiculopathy
4. cerebrovascular incidents

230. Types of analgesia that have been shown to be reversible by naloxone include
1. stimulation of periacqueductal grey matter
2. acupuncture
3. morphine
4. placebo

231. Valproate

1. is significantly more effective in the treatment of myoclonic seizures than in the treatment of atonic seizures
2. is significantly more effective than ethosuximide in the treatment of petit mal seizures
3. is significantly more effective than ethosuximide in the treatment of tonic clonic seizures
4. is significantly more effective than phenytoin in the treatment of partial seizures, although its use is limited by its high incidence of hepatotoxicity

232. Side effects of valproate include

1. alopecia
2. tremor
3. coagulopathy
4. rigidity

233. The serum level of the following may increase when given with valproate.

1. Phenytoin
2. Carbamazepine
3. Phenobarbital
4. Ethosuximide

234. Myasthenia gravis may be exacerbated by

1. quinidine
2. aminoglycosides
3. tetracycline
4. amantadine

235. The following may exacerbate myasthenia gravis through interference with presynaptic calcium ion fluxes.

1. Amantadine
2. Phenytoin
3. Procainamide
4. Chlorpromazine

Directions Summarized

(A) 1, 2, 3 only; **(B)** 1, 3 only; **(C)** 2, 4 only; **(D)** 4 only; **(E)** all

236. Benzodiazepines
1. are effective in treating status epilepticus
2. treat spasticity more effectively in patients with complete spinal cord transection than in those with incomplete spinal cord transection
3. bind far more frequently in the cerebellum than in the spinal cord
4. act directly on GABA receptors, with a direct GABA-mimetic effect

237. The following statements are true.
1. Baclofen is an effective treatment for patients with complete spinal cord transection
2. Dantrolene sodium is an effective treatment for patients with complete spinal cord transection
3. A significant complication of therapy with dantrolene sodium may be hepatic toxicity
4. Dantrolene sodium promotes the release of calcium ions from sarcoplasmic reticulum

238. Dystonia may complicate therapy with
1. levodopa
2. carbamazepine
3. phenothiazines
4. phenytoin

239. Propranolol
1. is the treatment of choice for benign essential tremor and will rapidly suppress this tremor when infused intraarterially
2. is a B adrenergic blocker which does not penetrate the blood-brain barrier
3. is quite effective in the treatment of cerebellar tremor
4. produces a clinical response which is unrelated to its plasma level in the treatment of benign essential tremor

240. Aspirin probably inhibits platelet aggregation by inhibiting

1. phospholipase A_2
2. prostacyclin synthetase
3. cyclic AMP
4. cyclo-oxygenase

4 NEUROPHYSIOLOGY

DIRECTIONS: Each of the questions or incomplete statements below is followed by a list of suggested answers or completions. Select the **one** that is best in each case.

241. The neuronal Na^+/K^+ pump
- **A.** is coupled to a cytoplasmic ATPase
- **B.** is activated by external Na^+
- **C.** is activated by internal K^+
- **D.** is regulated by changes in resting membrane potential
- **E.** is inhibited by digoxin

242. All of the following have an excitatory effect on the postsynaptic cell EXCEPT
- **A.** increased permeability to Ca^+
- **B.** slow increased permeability to Na^+
- **C.** decreased permeability to K^+
- **D.** increased permeability to K^+
- **E.** fast increased permeability to Na^+

243. Exocytotic release of vesicles at the synapse is most dependent upon
- **A.** Ca^+ influx
- **B.** K^+ influx
- **C.** Na^+ influx
- **D.** K^+ efflux
- **E.** none of the above

244. The ionic mechanism associated with the electrophysiologic action of GABA is

A. activation of a electrogenic Na^+ pump
B. opening of an ion channel for Cl^-
C. closing an ion channel for K^+
D. activating a voltage sensitive Na^+ channel
E. none of the above

245. The memory deficit characteristic of Korsakoff's syndrome can be produced by bilateral destruction of one of the following structures.

A. Parietal association cortex
B. Frontal association cortex
C. Hippocampus
D. Substantia innominata
E. None of the above

246. Identify the manner in which stimulus intensity is coded by tonic receptors.

A. Frequency of firing, since stronger stimuli can fire the axon earlier in the absolute refractory period
B. Frequency of firing, since stronger stimuli can fire the axon earlier in the relative refractory period
C. Frequency of firing, since stronger stimuli produce more rapid rates of depolarization toward threshold
D. Amplitude of action potential, due to the cable properties of axons
E. None of the above

247. Bilateral lesions of the lateral hypothalamus are associated with

A. aphasia
B. aphagia
C. hyperphagia
D. polyuria
E. hyposexuality

248. The electrical event associated with an increase in permeability just to K^+ is the

- **A.** action potential
- **B.** motoneuron hyperpolarizing afterpotential
- **C.** inhibitory postsynaptic potential
- **D.** excitatory postsynaptic potential

249. The equilibrium potential of Na^+ for mammalian motoneurons is

- **A.** +70 mV
- **B.** + 60 mV
- **C.** 0 mV
- **D.** -70 mV
- **E.** none of the above

250. The IPSP is associated with

- **A.** increased permeability to K^+
- **B.** increased permeability to Cl^-
- **C.** increased permeability to K^+ and Cl^-
- **D.** increased permeability to Na^+
- **E.** none of the above

251. Increasing the external concentration of Na^+

- **A.** hyperpolarizes a nerve cell during the resting state but leaves the peak voltage of the action potential unchanged
- **B.** depolarizes a nerve cell during the resting state but leaves the peak voltage of the action potential unchanged
- **C.** does not change the resting potential very much but decreases the amplitude of the action potential
- **D.** does not change the resting potential very much but increases the amplitude of the action potential

252. Since a given muscle cell can either twitch or remain silent, smooth, graded contractions require special mechanisms. Choose the one of the following which is NOT such a mechanism.

A. Increase in the rate of firing of a given motor unit, below the frequency of mechanical summation

B. Increase in the rate of firing of a given motor unit to the point that individual twitches are no longer separable

C. Increase in the number of active motor units

D. Increase in the number of muscle fibers in a motor unit

253. Local anesthetics placed on a muscle nerve in amounts too small to block large myelinated afferents

A. have no effect on motor function of that muscle

B. decrease motor activity in that muscle, since motor fibers are more sensitive to local anesthetics than are afferents of the same diameter

C. increase motor activity in that muscle

D. decrease motor activity in that muscle due to blockage of gamma motor fibers

E. none of the above

254. Choose the LEAST correct: Lesions of posterior parietal cortex of the nondominant hemisphere may give rise to the following symptoms.

A. Failure to groom the contralateral half of the body

B. Failure to complete the contralateral half of drawings

C. Failure to recognize the names of body parts

D. Failure to perceive a stimulus to the contralateral body half if the homologous ipsilateral area is stimulated simultaneously

E. Difficulty with paper and pencil constructions, e.g., "draw a cube"

255. Which of these statements is false?
- **A.** Most mammalian muscles contain both fast and slow fibers
- **B.** Slow fibers are "white" muscle
- **C.** Fast fibers are innervated by large motoneurons
- **D.** Fast fibers fatigue easily
- **E.** Fast fibers have low myoglobin content

256. Choose the property least characteristic of synaptic transmission.
- **A.** Undirectional conduction
- **B.** Ability to reproduce high rates of presynaptic firing
- **C.** Susceptibility to anoxia
- **D.** Plasticity

257. If the head is tilted to the right, reflex eye movements occur to
- **A.** shift the gaze to the left
- **B.** shift the gaze to the right
- **C.** produce convergence of the eyes
- **D.** rotate the eyes about their antero-posterior axis
- **E.** produce nystagmus

258. Comparing the compound action potential (CAP) recorded from an electrode near stimulating electrodes on the sciatic nerve to the CAP from a more distant electrode, which of the following is wrong?
- **A.** The peak of the alpha component is higher at the near electrode
- **B.** The peak of the alpha component is higher at the far electrode
- **C.** The alpha and beta peaks are more greatly separated at the far electrode
- **D.** The conduction velocity of both components can be measured
- **E.** None of the above

259. A motor unit comprises

A. the set of alpha motor neurons to a given muscle
B. the set of alpha and gamma motor neurons to a given muscle
C. the set of alpha motor neurons to a given muscle and the muscle fibers which they innervate
D. the set of muscle fibers innervated by a single motor neuron plus that neuron
E. the neuromuscular junction

260. Stimulation of group Ia afferents from an extensor muscle

A. enhances excitability of heteronymous synergists
B. enhances excitability of heteronymous antagonists
C. reduces excitability of the muscle whose nerve is stimulated
D. leads to melting of decerebrate rigidity
E. none of the above

261. The decrease in the size of the monosynaptic reflex during presynaptic inhibition is due to

A. decreased permeability of the motor neuron to Na^+
B. refractoriness of the presynaptic ending
C. decreased transmitter release by the presynaptic ending
D. hyperpolarization of the presynaptic ending

262. Identify the ultastructural homologue of the miniature end plate potential.

A. Synaptosomes
B. Synaptic vesicles
C. Desmosomes
D. Neurotubules
E. Neurofilaments

263. Choose the LEAST correct: The Kluver–Bucy syndrome, produced by bilateral temporal lobectomy, includes

A. hypersexuality
B. excessive oral behavior
C. increased exploratory behavior
D. increased fearfulness

264. Following spinal transection in humans
- **A.** flexor reflexes return earlier than extensor reflexes
- **B.** extensor reflexes return earlier than flexor reflexes
- **C.** extensor and flexor reflexes return at substantially the same time
- **D.** sweating is a frequent response to strong stimulation shortly after the trauma
- **E.** spasticity is a very early response

265. Choose the INCORRECT answer: Stimulation of the bulbar inhibitory reticular formation leads to
- **A.** reduction of decerebrate rigidity
- **B.** decreased gamma efferent discharge
- **C.** increased firing of group Ia afferents
- **D.** decreased size of the patellar reflex
- **E.** none of the above

266. Choose the INCORRECT answer: Fibers from the olfactory bulb project to
- **A.** the opposite olfactory bulb
- **B.** the prepyriform area and amygdaloid complex
- **C.** the olfactory tubercle
- **D.** the intralaminar nuclei of the thalamus
- **E.** the limbic system

267. In the precentral area
- **A.** cells which activate a given muscle are located in a cluster, with some overlap with cell clusters activating other muscles
- **B.** cells which activate extensors at a given joint are mingled together, but separate from those which activate flexors at the same joint
- **C.** cells which activate a given muscle are located in a very small area, with no overlap occurring among the various groups
- **D.** the number of cells activating a given muscle shows no correlation with the function of the muscle

268. In an electron photomicrograph of a cross section of the A band of striated muscle, it is seen that each myosin filament is surrounded by
- **A.** 4 actin filaments
- **B.** 6 actin filaments
- **C.** 8 actin filaments
- **D.** variable numbers of actin filaments
- **E.** none of the above

269. The shape of the frequency-threshold curve (audiometer curve) is determined primarily by
- **A.** the structure of the external auditory canal and the ossicles
- **B.** the structure of the organ of Corti
- **C.** neural connections at the medullary level
- **D.** neural connections at the cortical level

270. In general, long-lasting cortical events, such as the primary evoked potential, the recruiting response and the augmenting response are thought to be due to
- **A.** highly synchronized barrages of action potentials in thalamocortical afferents
- **B.** summated effects of the EPSPs and IPSPs induced in cortical neurons by the afferent barrage
- **C.** electrical events unrelated to the behavior of neurons
- **D.** pathological processes not seen in normal animals

271. Identify the one of the following nerve cell types not found in the retina.
- **A.** Horizontal cell
- **B.** Amacrine cell
- **C.** Granule cell
- **D.** Ganglion cell
- **E.** None of the above

272. Select the best description of the receptive field of retinal ganglion cells.

A. A circular region of retina, strongly excitatory toward the middle and weakly excitatory near the periphery

B. A circular region of retina, inhibitory except for a bar-shaped excitatory region, usually on a diameter

C. A circular region of retina, excitatory or inhibitory with a surrounding area which has the opposite effect of the center

D. A bar-shaped region of retina, excitatory, with an inhibitory surround

273. According to Hubel and Wiesel, simple visual cortical cells are sensitive to

A. diffuse areas of light on the retina

B. small spots of light anywhere on the retina

C. light bars oriented at particular angles anywhere on the retina

D. light bars oriented at particular angles, located on very restricted retinal areas

E. A and C

274. The centrifugal auditory pathway, called the bundle of Rasmussen

A. has not been shown to have any demonstrable function

B. has its effect by action of the small middle ear muscles on the ossicles

C. decreases auditory threshold

D. can be shown to decrease the size of auditory evoked potentials

E. none of the above

DIRECTIONS: For each of the questions or incomplete statements below, **one or more** of the answers or completions given is correct. Select

(A) if only 1, 2, and 3 are correct
(B) if only 1 and 3 are correct
(C) if only 2 and 4 are correct
(D) if only 4 is correct
(E) if all are correct

---

275. Agents that act on the Na^+ - channel include

1. lidocaine
2. veratradine
3. tetrodotoxin
4. tetraethylammonium

DIRECTIONS: Each group of questions below consists of a list of lettered headings followed by a list of numbered words or statements. For **each** numbered word or statement, select the **one** lettered heading that is most closely associated with it. Each lettered heading may be selected once, more than once, or not at all.

Electrical stimulation of certain brain areas can produce specific results. Match the brain areas below with the effect you would expect stimulation there to produce. Use each choice once only.

A. Animal will perform a learned task to obtain stimulation (self-stimulation)
B. Augmenting response recorded from motor cortex
C. Inhibition of spinal reflexes
D. Decreased food intake
E. Recruiting response recorded from cortex
F. Sexual responses (masturbation + autonomic effects)
G. Activation of cortical EEG
H. "Melting" of decerebrate rigidity
I. Amorphous visual sensations
J. Increased food intake

276. Ventromedial nucleus of hypothalamus
277. Lateral region of hypothalamus
278. Lateral geniculate body
279. Ventrolateral nucleus of thalamus
280. Centrum median nucleus of thalamus
281. Cingulate gyrus
282. Septal nuclei
283. Cerebellar cortex
284. Mesencephalic reticular formation
285. Medullary reticular formation

5 NEUROCHEMISTRY

DIRECTIONS: Each of the questions or incomplete statements below is followed by a list of suggested answers or completions. Select the **one** that is best in each case.

---

286. The rate limiting step for acetylcholine synthesis is
- **A.** choline acetylation
- **B.** choline phosphorylation
- **C.** choline supply
- **D.** acetyl-CoA synthesis
- **E.** none of the above

287. Cell bodies of neurons using beta-endorphin as the neurotransmitter are located in the
- **A.** substantia nigra
- **B.** arcuate nucleus of the hypothalamus
- **C.** periacqueductal gray matter
- **D.** dorsal horn of the spinal cord
- **E.** amygdala

288. All of the following peptides are derived from a common precursor EXCEPT
- **A.** beta endorphin
- **B.** ACTH
- **C.** cholecystikinin
- **D.** melanocyte-stimulating hormone
- **E.** beta-lipotropin

289. The brain utilizes approximately what percentage of total body O_2 consumption?
- **A.** 10%
- **B.** 15%
- **C.** 20%
- **D.** 30%
- **E.** None of the above

290. Apart from glucose, the only other sugar that the brain can utilize directly is
- **A.** maltose
- **B.** lactose
- **C.** galactose
- **D.** mannose
- **E.** none of the above

291. All of the following substances stimulate the rate of glycolysis in the brain EXCEPT
- **A.** NM_4^+
- **B.** K^+
- **C.** cyclic Amp
- **D.** ATP
- **E.** phosphate (inorganic)

292. N-acetylneuraminic acid is a
- **A.** sulfatide
- **B.** cerebroside
- **C.** ganglioside
- **D.** ceramide
- **E.** none of the above

293. Infants with Leigh's disease have a defect in the metabolism of which substance?
- **A.** Glycogen
- **B.** Acetyl Co A
- **C.** Thiamine
- **D.** Pyridoxine
- **E.** Cyanocobalamin

294. Major components of myelin include all EXCEPT
- **A.** cholesterol
- **B.** cerebroside
- **C.** lecithin
- **D.** sphingomyelin
- **E.** ethanolamine phosphatides

295. Termination of the action of catecholamines is mediated primarily by
- **A.** MAO
- **B.** COMT
- **C.** dopamine-beta hydroxylase
- **D.** reuptake
- **E.** amino acid decarboxylase

296. LSD-25 structurally resembles
- **A.** dopamine
- **B.** serotonin
- **C.** epinephrine
- **D.** norephinephrine
- **E.** none of the above

297. Triglycerides are found in large quantities
- **A.** in the pons
- **B.** in grey matter
- **C.** in white matter
- **D.** in the cerebellum
- **E.** nowhere in the brain

298. Patients with McArdle's disease have a deficiency of
- **A.** creatinine kinase
- **B.** acid maltase
- **C.** phosphofructokinase
- **D.** phosphorylase (glucose-6-phosphatase)
- **E.** none of the above

299. Cerebral respiratory rate first is decreased when the blood glucose falls to
- **A.** 10 mg %
- **B.** 20 mg %
- **C.** 50 mg %
- **D.** 35 mg %
- **E.** none of the above

300. The main oxidizable substrate of the human brain is
- **A.** glutamate
- **B.** albumin
- **C.** glucose
- **D.** fructose
- **E.** none of the above

DIRECTIONS: For each of the questions or incomplete statements below, **one or more** of the answers or completions given is correct. Select
- **(A)** if only 1, 2, and 3 are correct
- **(B)** if only 1 and 3 are correct
- **(C)** if only 2 and 4 are correct
- **(D)** if only 4 is correct
- **(E)** if all are correct

---

301. Infusion of dopamine into the third ventricle causes increased plasma levels of
1. FSH
2. TSH
3. LH
4. prolactin

302. Peptides that have been shown to act as neurotransmitters or neuromodulators include
1. vasopressin
2. cholecystikinin
3. vasoactive intestinal peptide
4. substance P

303. Criteria needed to categorize a neurotransmitter include
1. substance is present in nerve terminals
2. substance can cross the blood-brain barrier
3. a mechanism exists to inactivate the substance
4. only one neurotransmitter is released by a given neuron

304. Patients with malignant hyperpyrexia
1. have a defect in the heat-dissipating mechanism in the hypothalamus
2. have abnormal muscle biopsies
3. usually recover spontaneously
4. are sensitive to caffeine

305. Dopaminergic projections include
1. tuberoinfundibular
2. mesocortical
3. nigrostriatal
4. septo-hippocampal

306. Which of the following enzymes are involved in norepinephrine synthesis?
1. Aromatic acid decarboxylase
2. Phenylethanolamine N-methyltransferase
3. Tyrosine hydroxylose
4. Monoamine oxidase

307. Which of the following neurotransmitters have their synaptic action terminated by a reuptake mechanism?
1. Dopamine
2. Serotonin
3. Norepinephrine
4. Acetylcholine

308. Benzodiazepines modulate the synaptic actions of
1. glycine
2. dopamine
3. acetylcholine
4. GABA

DIRECTIONS: Each set of lettered headings below is followed by a list of numbered words or phrases. For each numbered word or phrase select

- **(A)** if the item is associated with A only
- **(B)** if the item is associated with B only
- **(C)** if the item is associated with both A and B
- **(D)** if the item is associated with neither A nor B

A. Inhibitory neurotransmitters
B. Excitatory neurotransmitters
C. Both
D. Neither

309. GABA
310. Glutamate
311. Glycine
312. Aspartate

Match

A. Hexosaminidase deficiency
B. Sphingomyelinase deficiency
C. Both
D. Neither

313. Tay-Sachs disease
314. Gaucher's disease
315. Cherry-red spot
316. Five types are known
317. Niemann-Pick disease
318. Sandhoff's disease
319. Hepatosplenomegaly

A. Metachromatic leukodystrophy
B. Krabbe's disease
C. Both
D. Neither

320. Galactocerebrosidase deficiency
321. Arylsulfatase A deficiency
322. Peripheral nervous system affected
323. Disease of white matter

A. B-endorphin
B. Enkephalin
C. Both
D. Neither

324. Widely distributed in brain and spinal cord
325. Found in the gastrointestinal tract
326. High concentrations found in the pituitary gland
327. Short-lived analgesia
328. Anti-diuretic effects
329. Increase release of substance P in the spinal cord

DIRECTIONS: Each group of questions below consists of a list of lettered headings followed by a list of numbered words or statements. For **each** numbered word or statement, select the **one** lettered heading that is most closely associated with it. Each lettered heading may be selected once, more than once, or not at all.

Match the substance with the area with which it is primarily associated.

A. Paraventricular nucleus
B. Periacqueductal grey
C. Arcuate nucleus
D. Suprachiasmatic nucleus
E. Ventromedial nucleus (of the hypothalamus)

330. Beta-endorphin
331. Oxytocin
332. Vasopressin
333. Substance P

Match the sarcomere component with the most appropriate statement.

A. Contains enzyme activity
B. Found in the Z band
C. Found in the I band
D. Confers Ca^{++} dependence

334. Myosin
335. Actin
336. Tropomyosin

Match the neurotoxin with its most characteristic clinical effect.

A. Manganese
B. Lead
C. Carbon tetrachloride
D. Acrylamide
E. Mercury

337. Optic atrophy
338. Parkinsonism
339. Wrist drop
340. Ataxia

Match the substance with its mode of action on the neuromuscular junction.

A. Increased ACh release
B. Decreased ACh release
C. Blockade of ACh receptors
D. Destruction of ACh receptors

341. Botulinum toxin
342. Alpha-bungaro toxin
343. Black widow spider venom

Match the vitamin deficiency with its clinical or pathologic correlate.

A. Central chromatolysis
B. Lower seizure threshold
C. Demyelination
D. "Burning foot" syndrome

344. B-12
345. Niacin
346. Pantothenic acid
347. Pyridoxine

Match the ion with its effect on the neuron.

A. Ca^{++}
B. Na^{+}
C. K^{+}

348. Critical for exocytosis
349. Increase in permeability depolarizes cell
350. High intracellular concentration

6 DIAGNOSTIC NEUROLOGY

DIRECTIONS: Each of the questions or incomplete statements below is followed by a list of suggested answers or completions. Select the **one** that is best in each case.

---

351. Myelographic signs of chronic herniated disc include all EXCEPT

A. hourglass deformity of dye column
B. "double" contour on prone films
C. tenting of the dura
D. complete block of dye column
E. none of the above

352. Meningiomas most often produce enlargement of which artery?

A. Anterior cerebral
B. Middle cerebral
C. Middle meningeal
D. Internal carotid
E. Superficial temporal

353. Characteristics of optic gliomas include

A. atrophic optic canal
B. rounding of sella turcica
C. "double" optic foramina
D. frequently associated with neurofibromatosis
E. none of the above

354. Suture separation in the skull and a wide band of heavy density at the ends of long bone shafts on x-ray should suggest

A. hyperparathyroidism
B. fibrous dysplasia
C. lead poisoning
D. rickets
E. arsenic poisoning

355. The tumor most often causing ballooning of the sella is

A. eosinophilic pituitary adenoma
B. basophilic pituitary adenoma
C. chromophobe pituitary adenoma
D. dorsum sella meningioma
E. craniopharyngioma

356. After denervation the first evidence of fibrillation in human muscle occurs within

A. 2 days
B. 14–21 days
C. 30–40 days
D. 80–90 days
E. none of the above

357. The most likely diagnosis in a patient with a bruit and destruction at the base of the petrous pyramid is

A. chordoma
B. acoustic neurinoma
C. glomus jugulare tumor
D. carcinoma
E. arteriovenous malformation

358. The normal motor conduction velocity of a human peripheral nerve when tested by electromyography is

A. 10–20 meters per second
B. 20–30 meters per second
C. 40–60 meters per second
D. none of the above

359. Cloudlike, homogenous calcification in skull x-ray favors the diagnosis of

A. oligodendroglioma
B. meningioma
C. aneurysm
D. subdural hematoma
E. Sturge-Weber syndrome

360. On skull x-ray one finds hyperostosis, increased vascularity, and calcification. The diagnosis is

A. glioblastoma
B. oligodendroglioma
C. dermoid
D. meningioma
E. fibrous dysplasia
F. hyperostosis frontalis interna

361. Enlargement of the optic foramen is seen in

A. meningioma of the optic canal
B. neurofibromatosis
C. optic nerve glioma
D. ophthalamic artery aneurysm
E. any of the above

362. Posterior and upwards displacement of the anterior inferior cerebellar artery should suggest

A. pontine glioma
B. cerebellar astrocytoma
C. cerebellopontine angle tumor
D. clivus chordoma
E. medulloblastoma

363. On cerebral angiography one notes medial displacement of the anterior choroidal artery. One should suspect primarily

A. subfalcial herniation
B. brain stem tumor
C. anterior hippocampal herniation
D. cerebellar tonsillar herniation
E. subfrontal mass

364. Absence of the sphenoid wing is most commonly seen in
- **A.** tuberous sclerosis
- **B.** Von Recklinghausen's disease
- **C.** craniopharyngioma
- **D.** porencephalic cyst
- **E.** suprasellar meningioma

365. Arterial spasm on angiography may be seen in
- **A.** syphilis
- **B.** amphetamine abuse
- **C.** atrial myxoma
- **D.** polyarteritis nodosa
- **E.** any of the above

366. The most common tumor to produce suprasellar calcification is
- **A.** chromophobe adenoma
- **B.** optic nerve glioma
- **C.** craniopharyngioma
- **D.** aneurysm
- **E.** clivus chordoma

367. The least useful radiological sign of an intravertebral tumor on plain spine films is
- **A.** enlargement of the intravertebral foramen
- **B.** spondylolisthesis
- **C.** thinning of the lamina
- **D.** calcification within the tumor
- **E.** scalloping of the posterior margins of the vertebral bodies

368. Among the glioma group of tumors, the most common to calcify is
- **A.** ependymoma
- **B.** medulloblastoma
- **C.** oligodendroglioma
- **D.** astrocytoma
- **E.** ganglioglioma

369. A characteristic EEG response to barbiturates is
A. bursts of 20–24 c/s activity
B. bursts of rapid eye movements
C. biparietal sharp waves
D. increased alpha activity
E. none of the above

370. In the differential diagnosis of multiple intracerebral calcifications, one should not consider likely
A. toxoplasmosis
B. metastatic brain abscesses
C. cytomegalic inclusion disease
D. cysticercosis
E. tuberous sclerosis

371. The presence of K complexes on the EEG indicates the presence of
A. astrocytoma
B. meningioma
C. thalamic tumor
D. phenothiazine toxicity
E. none of the above

372. A clear area of bone destruction in the skull surrounded by sclerotic bone is seen. The least likely lesion is
A. epidermoid tumor
B. cavernous hemangioma
C. osteoma
D. eosinophilic granuloma
E. localized fibrous dysplasia

373. Upon performing a lumbar puncture one obtained cerebrospinal fluid which was clear and xanthochromic under increased pressure. The most likely diagnosis is
A. Froin's syndrome
B. traumatic lumbar puncture
C. very recently ruptured aneurysm
D. chronic subdural hematoma
E. inadequately treated meningitis

374. The most frequent cause of diminished density of the skull is

A. parathyroid disease
B. aging
C. increased pressure
D. hypervitaminosis D
E. Cushing's syndrome

375. The most common intraventricular tumors are

A. meningiomas
B. gliomas
C. choroid plexus papillomas
D. lipomas
E. colloid cysts

376. Generally a "rounded shift" of the anterior cerebral artery on angiography indicates a tumor in the

A. anterior frontal lobe
B. parietal lobe
C. posterior temporal lobe
D. occipital lobe
E. none of the above

377. All of the following are classified as pseudoepileptiform patterns EXCEPT

A. 6 Hz spike and slow wave
B. small sharp spikes
C. 14 and 6 Hz positive bursts
D. independent multifocal spikes
E. none of the above

378. The H response

A. reflects polysynaptic reflex activity
B. is useful for assessing proximal peripheral nerve dysfunction
C. occurs maximally with supramaximal stimulation of the motor nerve
D. appears after the M response is generated
E. none of the above

379. Normal sensory action potential in a patient with sensory loss
- **A.** may indicate a poor prognosis for recovery because preganglionic damage precludes regeneration of sensory fibers
- **B.** indicates a good prognosis for recovery
- **C.** is not associated with traumatic root avulsion
- **D.** should not be seen in patients with syringomyelia
- **E.** may accompany traumatic plexus injury

380. Temporal dispersion
- **A.** is more pronounced in sensory than motor fibers
- **B.** affects the muscle response more than the nerve action potential, when no nerve pathology is present
- **C.** produces an action potential of increased amplitude and smaller duration
- **D.** is inversely proportional to the conduction distance
- **E.** none of the above

381. The blink reflex elicited by electrical stimulation of the supraorbital nerve is most often normal in
- **A.** trigeminal neuralgia
- **B.** pontine glioma
- **C.** Bell's palsy
- **D.** acoustic neuroma
- **E.** none of the above

382. A stimulus submaximal for the regular compound muscle action potential best elicits
- **A.** the M response
- **B.** the H reflex
- **C.** the F wave
- **D.** none of the above
- **E.** B and C

383. Nerve conduction velocity is faster
- **A.** at limb temperatures less than 34°C
- **B.** between ages 5 and 30
- **C.** in shorter patients than in taller patients
- **D.** in the distal segments than in the proximal segments
- **E.** B and C

384. Arachnoiditis following iophendylate myelography
- **A.** is radiographically apparent in as many as 67% of patients
- **B.** produces back pain and sacral and lumbar root dysfunction in as many as 67% of patients
- **C.** generally produces symptoms several years following myelography, symptoms which are difficult to distinguish from those produced by the patient's underlying condition
- **D.** should be treated surgically
- **E.** none of the above

385. Following metrizamide myelography
- **A.** EEG abnormalities may be seen in 10–35% of patients
- **B.** adhesive arachnoiditis is a well-reported complication
- **C.** dye entry into the intracranial cavity may be prevented by maintaining an upright position
- **D.** chronic reactions are more common than acute
- **E.** none of the above

386. Nerve conduction velocity will be slower in
- **A.** a 50-year-old man with limb temperature of 38°C
- **B.** a 20-year-old man with skin temperature of 28°C
- **C.** a 40-year-old man with a limb temperature of 36°C
- **D.** The age and temperature differences in these subjects will balance the differences produced in nerve conduction velocities, and all will have equal conduction velocities

387. The neurologic complications of arteriography include
- **A.** seizures in 5–10% of cases
- **B.** generalized brain edema in 2–5%
- **C.** transient cortical blindness in 0.3–1% of vertebral studies
- **D.** A and B
- **E.** none of the above

388. The neurologic complications of intravenous contrast dye administration

A. occur in more than 5% of patients with brain metastasis receiving dye for CT scan

B. include spinal seizures in patients with spinal cord AVM

C. occur in 5% of patients with spinal cord AVM

D. A and B

E. none of the above

389. The most common complication of iophendylate (pantopaque) myelography is

A. transverse myelopathy

B. fever

C. CSF pleocytosis

D. symptomatic adhesive arachnoiditis

E. none of the above

390. Visual evoked responses

A. are prolonged in Parkinson's disease due to associated degeneration of optic nerves

B. are prolonged in Parkinson's disease due to the associated dopaminergic deficiency

C. are prolonged in Parkinson's disease on a nutritional basis

D. should not be prolonged in uncomplicated Parkinson's disease

---

DIRECTIONS: For each of the questions or incomplete statements below, **one or more** of the answers or completions given is correct. Select

- **(A)** if only 1, 2, and 3 are correct
- **(B)** if only 1 and 3 are correct
- **(C)** if only 2 and 4 are correct
- **(D)** if only 4 is correct
- **(E)** if all are correct

---

391. BAERS
1. may be normal in barbiturate-induced coma
2. are less sensitive than VERs or SERs in indicating clinically silent lesions in patients with multiple sclerosis
3. have been shown to be somewhat useful in predicting the clinical outcome of coma
4. have been reported to be abnormal in some patients with Wilson's disease

392. The Martin-Gruber anomaly
1. is an anastomosis between median and ulnar nerves
2. is very rare, occurring in less than 1% of the population
3. causes a greater response to ulnar stimulation at the wrist than at the elbow
4. causes a greater response to ulnar nerve stimulation at the elbow than at the wrist

393. Normal finding in the EEG of adults over age 60 include
1. slowing of alpha frequency
2. increased beta activity
3. intermittent temporal slow waves
4. bilateral synchronous rhythmic delta activity

394. Beta rhythm may be increased in
1. diabetes insipidus
2. Valium ingestion
3. Cushing's disease
4. anxiety

Directions Summarized

(A) 1, 2, 3 only; **(B)** 1, 3 only; **(C)** 2, 4 only; **(D)** 4 only; **(E)** all

395. Normal EEG responses to hyperventilation
  1. are most common in older persons
  2. normally end 2 minutes after cessation of HV
  3. include bursts of asynchronous delta activity
  4. may be enhanced by hypoglycemia

DIRECTIONS: Each set of lettered headings below is followed by a list of numbered words or phrases. For each numbered word or phrase select
  (A) if the item is associated with A only
  (B) if the item is associated with B only
  (C) if the item is associated with both A and B
  (D) if the item is associated with neither A nor B

  A. Dopaminergic blockade
  B. Gabaergic blockade
  C. Both
  D. Neither

396. Alteration of VER latency
397. VER wave shape distortion

  A. VER
  B. BAER
  C. Both
  D. Neither

398. Latency increases with age after age 60
399. Latency is changed with decreased body temperature
400. Women have shorter latencies than men
401. May be normal in a patient with a normal clinical examination

DIRECTIONS: Each group of questions below consists of a list of lettered headings followed by a list of numbered words or statements. For **each** numbered word or statement, select the **one** lettered heading that is most closely associated with it. Each lettered heading may be selected once, more than once, or not at all.

A. Neuropraxia
B. Axonotmesis
C. Neurotmesis
D. All of the above
E. B and C

402. Nerve conduction ceases without structural change in the axon
403. Loss of axonal continuity with Wallerian degeneration of the distal segment
404. Demyelination may occur, and nerve conduction studies will demonstrate normal wave amplitude with decreased velocity
405. Stimulation distal to the lesion gives rise to no muscle action potentials if tested 4 days after injury

Match the EEG pattern with the stage of sleep with which it is associated.

A. Stage 1
B. Stage 2
C. Stage 3
D. REM

406. Sleep spindles
407. Delta activity
408. Theta activity
409. Sawtooth waves

Match the EEG pattern most often associated with the clinical picture.

- **A.** Jakob-Creutzfeldt
- **B.** Hepatic encephalopathy
- **C.** Postanoxic encephalopathy
- **D.** Brain tumor
- **E.** Sleep

410. Periodic lateralizing epileptiform discharge
411. Periodic sharp waves
412. Triphasic waves
413. Burst suppression
414. K-complexes

Match the radiological description and tumor.

- **A.** Extradural tumor
- **B.** Intramedullary tumor
- **C.** Extramedullary, intradural tumor

415. Partial obstruction to the flow of the contrast medium with fusiform cord enlargement
416. Sharp delineation of tumor margin with displacement of cord shadow
417. Conical narrowing of the column of contrast material in the vertebral canal

Match the following descriptions and diagnoses.

- **A.** Klippel Feil
- **B.** Platybasia
- **C.** Albers-Schonberg disease
- **D.** Trigonocephaly
- **E.** Hyperostosis frontalis interna

418. Localized increased thickness of the frontal bones
419. Increased density of skull bones
420. Congenital failure of segmentation of upper cervical vertebrae
421. Skull basal angle equals 160°
422. Premature synostosis of metopic suture

Match the following descriptions and diagnoses.

A. Bathrocephaly
B. Dandy-Walker syndrome
C. Increased intracranial pressure
D. Luckenschadel

423. Imperforate foramina of Luschka and Magendie with enlargement of posterior fossa
424. Irregular honeycomblike configuration of the bones of the skull
425. Overlap of upper aspect of occipital bone
426. Erosion of cortical bone of interior of sella turcica

Match the following descriptions and diagnoses.

A. Crouzon's disease
B. Scaphocephaly
C. Plagiocephaly
D. Acrocephalo-synactylism
E. Brachycephaly

427. Premature closure of the sagittal suture
428. Premature closure of the coronal and lambdoidal sutures
429. Generalized craniostenosis and hypoplasia of the facial bones
430. Premature fusion of one-half of the coronal suture
431. Premature synostosis with finger anomalies

Match the following angiographic description and probable diagnosis.

A. Subfrontal meningioma
B. Anterior temporal tumor
C. Ventricular dilatation
D. Acoustic neurinoma

432. Lateral displacement of thalamostriate vein with increased curvature
433. Elevated superior cerebellar artery
434. Elevation of anterior portion of sylvian triangle
435. Elevation of anterior cerebral artery

Match the following angiographic descriptions and tumors.

- **A.** Meningioma
- **B.** Glioblastoma
- **C.** Metastatic tumor
- **D.** Meningioma

436. Irregular beaded vessels in the periphery draining to deep veins
437. Supplied by branches of external carotid artery with sunburst appearance
438. Persistent homogenous tumor cloud
439. Multiple tumor stains supplied by single vessels

Match the following vascular displacements and tumor location.

- **A.** Parasagittal frontal
- **B.** Infra-Sylvian
- **C.** Frontal polar
- **D.** Occipital polar
- **E.** Thalamic

440. Rounded shift of anterior cerebral artery
441. Downward displacement of pericallosal artery
442. Elevation and medial displacement of middle cerebral branches
443. Forward displacement of Sylvian point
444. Normal middle cerebral artery and internal cerebral vein shifted

Match the diagnosis with the finding on a skull x-ray.

- **A.** Venous lakes
- **B.** Pacchonian granulations
- **C.** Metastatic cancer
- **D.** A and B
- **E.** None of the above

445. Lesion involves the inner and outer table
446. May exhibit depressions on the inner table of the skull
447. Lucency within the diploë

DIRECTIONS: Each group of questions below consists of figures alone or a figure with lettered components, followed by a list of numbered words or statements. For **each** numbered word or statement select the **one** figure or figure component that is most closely associated with it. Each figure or figure component may be selected once, more than once, or not at all.

Match the appropriate BAER wave shown in Fig. 6.1 to the anatomic correlate.

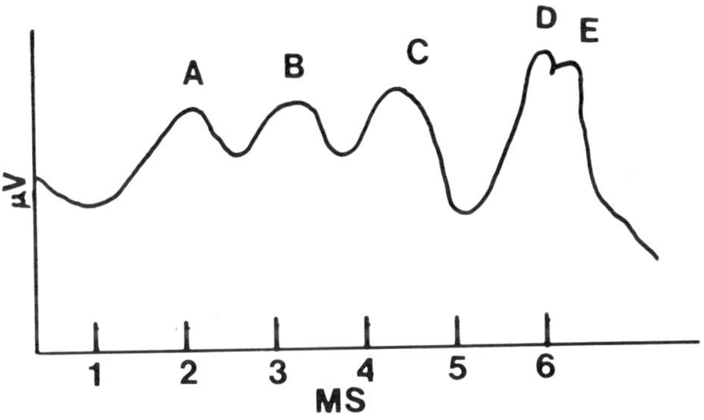

Figure 6.1

448. Lateral lemniscus
449. Cochlear nuclei
450. Inferior colliculus
451. Acoustic nerve
452. Superior olivary complex

Match the diagnoses with the scans shown in Figures 6.2–6.10.

A. Middle cerebral artery infarct
B. Pineal tumor
C. Putamenal hemorrhage
D. Multiple sclerosis
E. Thalamic glioma
F. Astrocytoma
G. Olivopontocerebellar atrophy
H. Normal
I. Wilson's disease
J. Normal pressure hydrocephalus

453. Figure 6.2
454. Figure 6.3
455. Figure 6.4
456. Figure 6.5
457. Figure 6.6
458. Figure 6.7
459. Figure 6.8
460. Figure 6.9
461. Figure 6.10

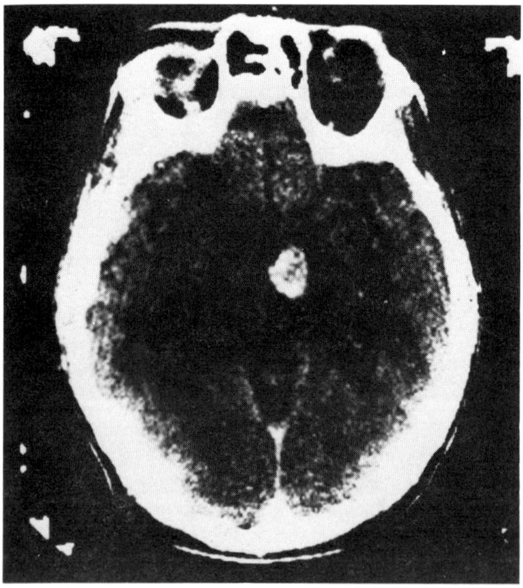

Figure 6.2

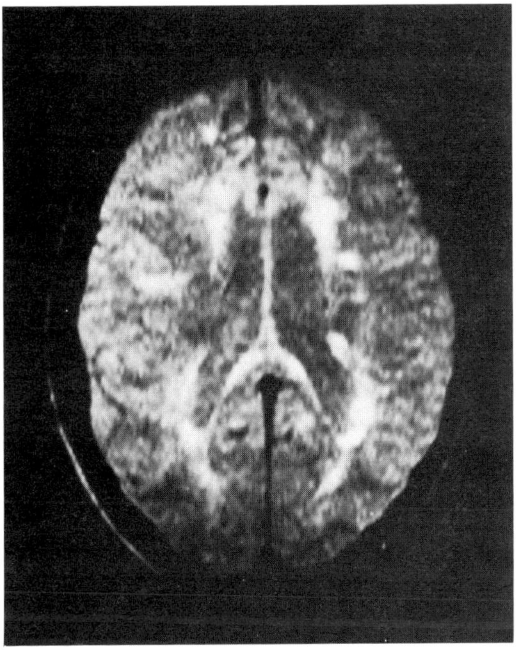

Figure 6.3

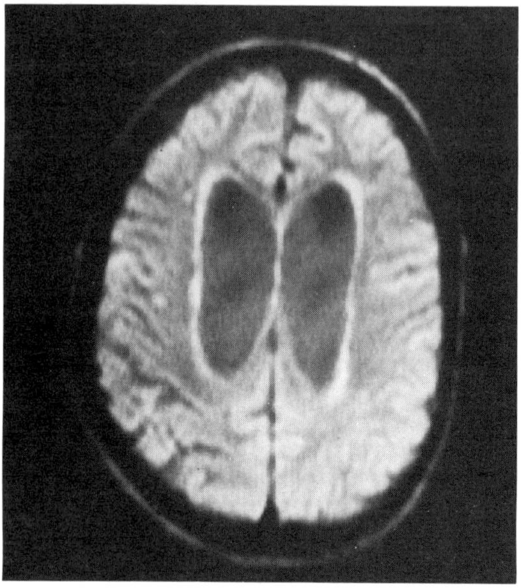

Figure 6.4

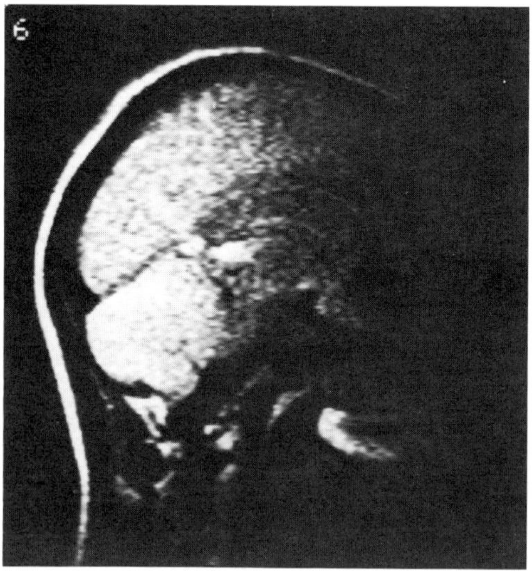

Figure 6.5

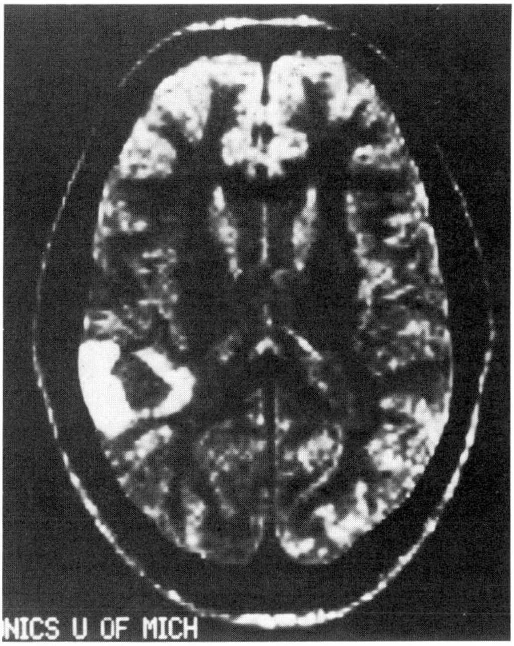

Figure 6.6

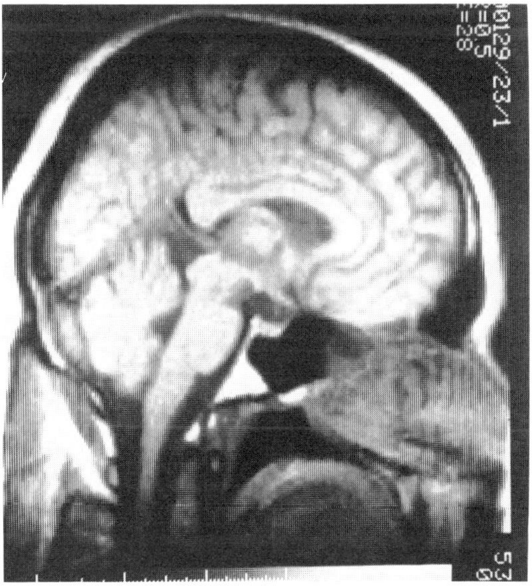

Figure 6.7

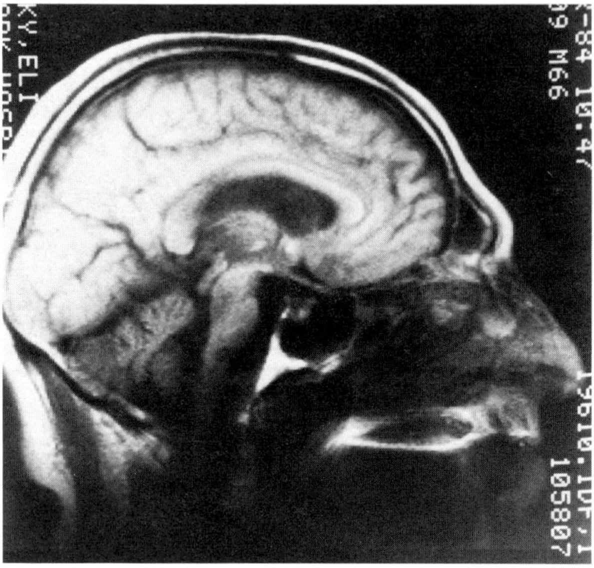

Figure 6.8

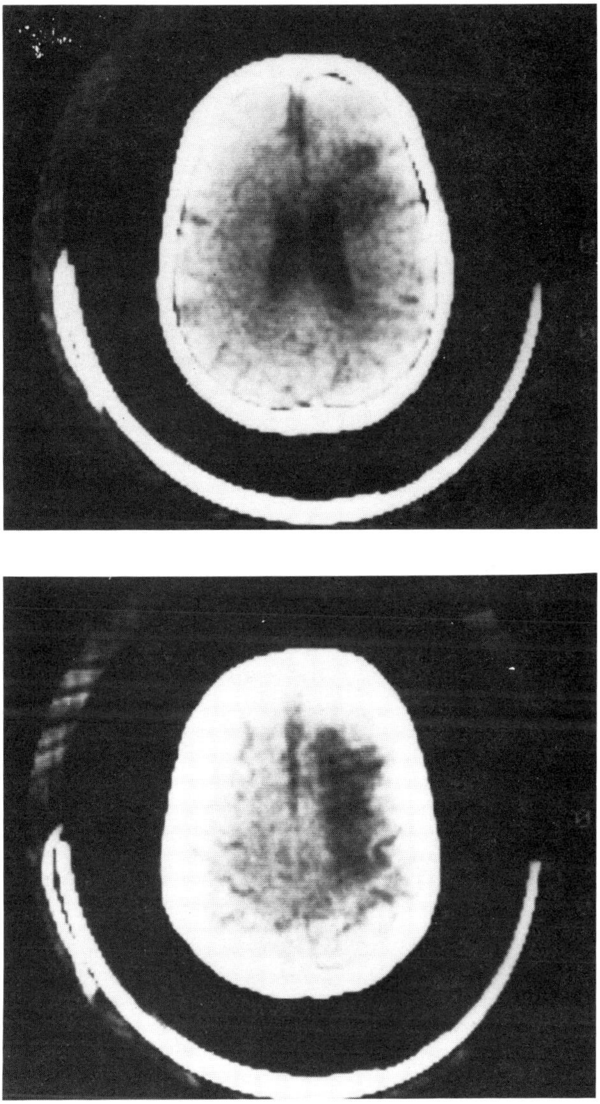

Figure 6.9

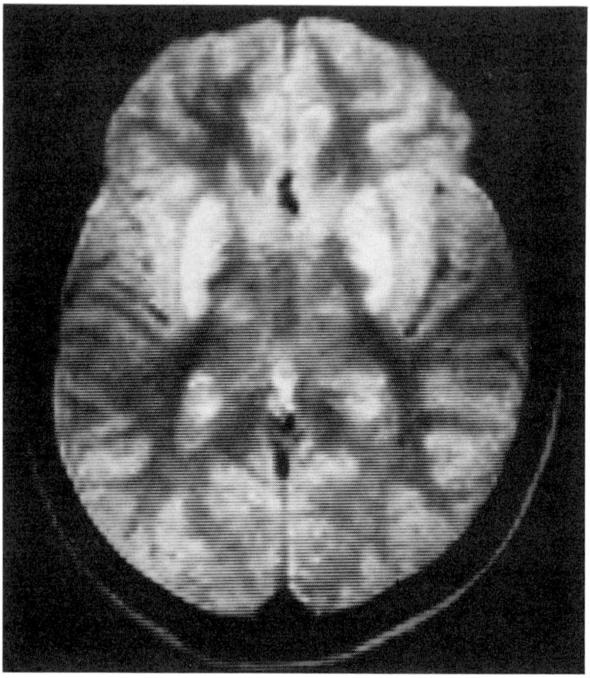

Figure 6.10

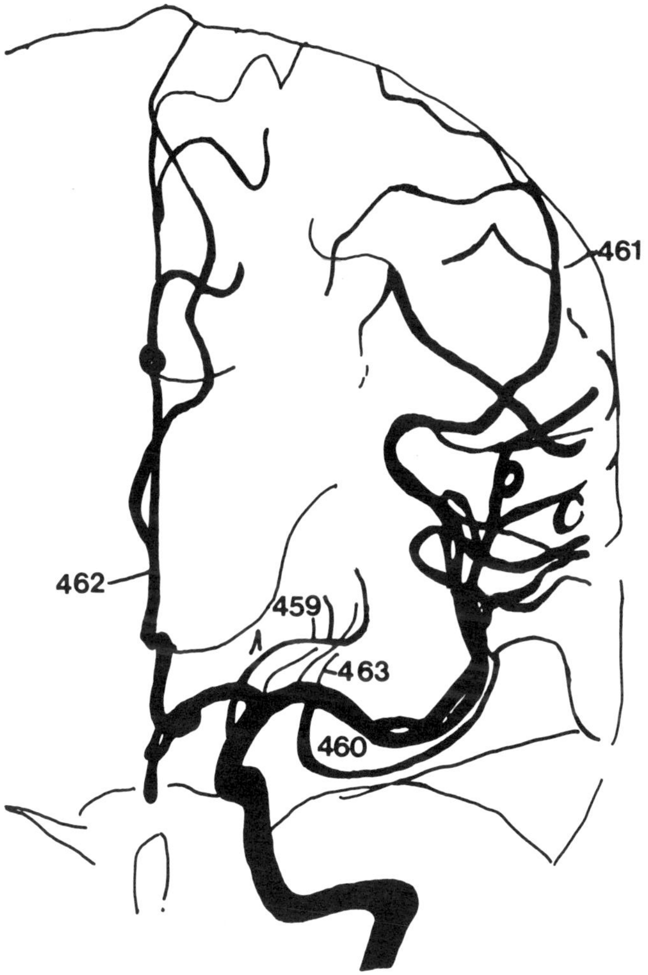

Figure 6.11

Match the blood vessels to the structures indicated in the angiogram depicted in Figure 6.11.

462. Anterior choroidal artery
463. Lenticulostriate artery
464. Middle cerebral artery
465. Pericallosal artery
466. Posterior parietal artery

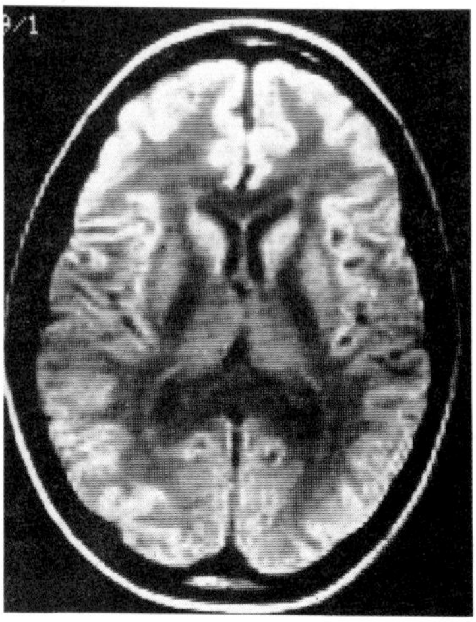

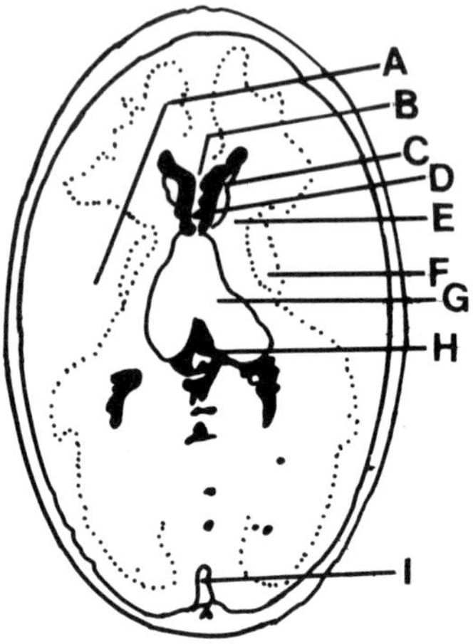

Figure 6.12

Match the structures with the lettered components shown in the MRI scan in Figure 6.12.

467. Putamen
468. Thalamus
469. Caudate
470. Internal capsule
471. Fornix
472. Dural sinus
473. Insular grey matter
474. Septum pellucidum
475. Third ventricle

7 PEDIATRIC CLINICAL NEUROLOGY

DIRECTIONS: Each of the questions or incomplete statements below is followed by a list of suggested answers or completions. Select the **one** that is best in each case.

---

476. At age three years a normal child
- **A.** can stand on one foot
- **B.** can tell right from left foot
- **C.** has extensor plantar responses
- **D.** has developed good tonic neck reflexes
- **E.** has lost the opticokinetic nystagmus

477. A two-year-old child with progressive gait difficulty, absent tendon reflexes, elevated spinal fluid protein, and urinary granules staining brown with toluidine blue should be diagnosed as
- **A.** Schilder's
- **B.** metachromatic leukodystrophy
- **C.** spongy degeneration
- **D.** diffuse sclerosis
- **E.** cerebral palsy

478. Eczema, blonde hair, blue eyes, and mental retardation are characteristic of
A. phenylketonuria
B. cretinism
C. tuberous sclerosis
D. mongolism
E. toxoplasmosis

479. The least common organism in childhood purulent meningitis is
A. meningococcus
B. H. influenza
C. pneumococcus
D. E. coli
E. A. aerogenes

480. The most common organism in posttraumatic meningitis is
A. staphylococcus
B. meningococcus
C. pneumococcus
D. streptococcus
E. H. influenza

481. The most common causative organism of meningitis between one and four years is
A. staphylococcus
B. meningococcus
C. pneumococcus
D. E. coli
E. H. influenza

482. In acute purulent meningitis the cerebrospinal fluid is almost never
A. opalescent
B. clear
C. cloudy
D. purulent
E. under increased pressure

483. Select the cerebrospinal fluid formula for acute purulent meningitis.

A. 25 Polys/Cu. mm; Protein 45 mg%; Sugar 50 mg %
B. 250 Polys/Cu. mm; Protein 45 mg %; Sugar 50 mg%
C. 250 Monos/Cu. mm; Protein 450 mg %; Sugar 50 mg %
D. 2500 Polys/Cu. mm; Protein 450 mg %; Sugar 50 mg %
E. 2500 Polys/Cu. mm; Protein 450 mg %; Sugar 10 mg %

484. The lumbar puncture revealed opalescent cerebrospinal fluid under increased pressure. The most likely diagnosis is

A. subarachnoid hemorrhage
B. traumatic puncture
C. tuberculous meningitis
D. normal but tense patient
E. brain tumor

485. Select the most likely cerebrospinal fluid formula in partially treated purulent meningitis.

A. 120 Polys/Cu. mm; Protein 40 mg %; Sugar 60 mg %
B. 1200 Polys/Cu. mm; Protein 40 mg %; Sugar 60 mg %
C. 1200 Monos/Cu. mm; Protein 30 mg %; Sugar 60 mg %
D. 120 Monos/Cu. mm; Protein 100 mg %; Sugar 20 mg %
E. 12,000 Polys/Cu. mm; Protein 40 mg %; Sugar 60 mg %

486. Select the most likely cerebrospinal formula in a patient with a localized brain abscess.
A. Normal pressure; 2 Monos/Cu. mm; Protein 40 mg %
B. Increased pressure; 20 Monos/Cu. mm; Protein 140 mg %
C. Increased pressure; 2000 Polys/Cu. mm; Protein 40 mg %
D. Normal pressure; 30 Monos/Cu. mm; Protein 20 mg %
E. Normal pressure; 2500 Polys/Cu. mm; Protein 400 mg %

487. In the differential diagnosis of tuberculous meningitis the most troublesome question is
A. brain tumor
B. subarachnoid hemorrhage
C. inadequately treated purulent meningitis
D. subdural hematoma
E. viral encephalitis

488. If the cerebrospinal fluid contained 400 mononuclear cells/Cu. mm and sugar 20 mg %, which is the most improbable condition present?
A. Torula meningitis
B. Yeast meningitis
C. Cryptococcal meningitis
D. Tuberculous meningitis
E. Acute staphylococcal meningitis

489. The organisms most commonly producing localized infections of the nervous system are
A. H. influenza, E. coli, and meningococci
B. H. influenza and E. coli
C. staphylococci, streptococci, and pneumococci
D. staphylococci, pneumococci, and meningococci
E. staphylococci, streptococci, and H. influenza

490. Fever, confusion, exophthalmos, chemosis, and extra-ocular muscle palsies in a child should cause one to diagnose

A. sphenoid ridge tumor
B. craniopharyngioma
C. septic cavernous sinus thrombosis
D. temporal lobe abscess
E. infraclinoid aneurysm

491. Fever, no nuchal rigidity, the occurrence of bilateral neurologic signs appearing first on one side and then on the other should cause one to suspect

A. parasagittal meningioma
B. cerebral abscess
C. cerebral embolus
D. sagittal sinus thrombosis
E. mucormycosis

492. Posterior fossa tumors constitute what percentage of intracranial tumors in pediatrics?

A. 95%
B. 65%
C. 45%
D. 30%
E. 5%

493. The commonest extraocular palsy in brain tumors in childhood is

A. unilateral external rectus
B. unilateral ptosis
C. unilteral internal rectus
D. bilateral internal rectus
E. bilateral external rectus

494. The commonest symptom of increased intracranial pressure in childhood is

A. blurred vision
B. stupor
C. vomiting
D. ataxia
E. double vision

495. Headache as a symptom of brain tumor in childhood is usually worse
- **A.** after school
- **B.** after dinner
- **C.** after retiring at night
- **D.** after arising in the morning
- **E.** after lunch

496. In a child, visual disturbances, diabetes insipidus, and retardation of growth should cause one to suspect
- **A.** pituitary adenoma
- **B.** craniopharyngioma
- **C.** subdural hematoma
- **D.** medulloblastoma
- **E.** retinoblastoma

497. In a child, headache, vomiting, ataxia, nystagmus and limitation of neck movements cause one to suspect
- **A.** craniopharyngioma
- **B.** medulloblastoma
- **C.** optic nerve glioma
- **D.** subdural hematoma
- **E.** frontal lobe astrocytoma

498. The more likely diagnosis in a child with headache, unilateral dysmetria, and papilledema is
- **A.** craniopharyngioma
- **B.** medulloblastoma
- **C.** cerebellar astrocytoma
- **D.** cerebral ependymoma
- **E.** pinealoma

499. Medulloblastomas usually arise in the
- **A.** thalamus
- **B.** basal ganglia
- **C.** cerebellar hemisphere
- **D.** roof of the fourth ventricle
- **E.** floor of the third ventricle

500. The following tumor is uncommon in childhood
A. glioblastoma
B. pontine glioma
C. medulloblastoma
D. optic nerve glioma
E. cerebellar astrocytoma

501. Progressive unilateral proptosis and decreasing visual acuity in a child should lead to the diagnosis of
A. optic nerve glioma
B. craniopharyngioma
C. sphenoid ridge meningioma
D. pinealoma
E. carotid cavernous fistula

502. In an infant with congestive heart failure, hydrocephalus, and convulsions one should suspect
A. perinatal cerebral abscess
B. subacute bacterial endocarditis
C. vein of Galen malformation
D. mongolism
E. cerebral angioma

503. The most common cause of intracranial hemorrhage in childhood is
A. intracranial aneurysm
B. trauma
C. blood dyscrasia
D. glomerulonephritis
E. liver disease

504. Two days after a fractured femur a child experiences confusion, hemiparesis, fever, and blood-tinged sputum. One should suspect
A. metastatic cerebral abscess
B. associated subdural hematoma
C. cerebral fat embolism
D. traumatic cerebral thrombosis
E. cortical contusion

505. Focal seizures, periodic migrainoid headaches, and subarachnoid hemorrhage in a teenager would indicate the presence of

A. vein of Galen malformation
B. Sturge Weber syndrome
C. idiopathic epilepsy
D. cerebral arteriovenous malformation
E. ruptured carotid aneurysm

506. A two-year-old child with dilated conjunctival blood vessels, recurrent infections, and ataxia most likely has

A. ataxia telangiectasia
B. Friedreich's ataxia
C. ataxia cerebral palsy
D. dentate cerebellar ataxia
E. Bassen-Kornzweig's syndrome

507. A six-year-old child with retinitis pigmentosa, cerebellar ataxia, pes cavus, scoliosis, and acanthocytosis most likely has

A. ataxia telangiectasia
B. Friedreich's ataxia
C. Refsum's syndrome
D. juvenile lipidosis
E. none of the above

508. Scoliosis, pes cavus, retinitis pigmentosa, and high arched palate are stigmata of

A. abetalipoproteinemia
B. syringomyelia
C. infantile lipidosis
D. juvenile lipidosis
E. cerebral palsy

509. A teenaged child had slowly progressive weakness and wasting in the extremities. There was pes cavus, distal sensory loss, and absent tendon reflexes. The diagnosis is most likely

A. Guillain-Barré
B. hypertrophic interstitial polyneuritis
C. diabetic polyneuritis
D. hereditary sensory neuropathy
E. Riley-Day syndrome

510. A four-year-old child developed vomiting, diarrhea, headache, and abdominal pain a few hours after ingesting an unknown liquid. Three days later confusion and convulsions developed. After a week, there was a motor neuropathy. The liquid most likely contained

A. lead salts
B. arsenicals
C. thallium salts
D. organic phosphorus compounds
E. mercury salts

511. A ten-year-old boy complained of gait difficulties. There was a family history of a similar disorder. On examination there was hyperreflexia and Babinski signs only. A likely diagnosis is

A. Levy-Roussy syndrome
B. Werdnig-Hoffman syndrome
C. familial spastic paraplegia
D. Friedreich's ataxia
E. Duchenne's dystrophy

512. A two-year-old child had a history of irritability, failure to thrive, motor regression, and then became confused. On examination of the blood, there was some anemia, and the test for urinary coproporphyrin III was positive. A diagnosis of the following should be made

A. chronic arsenical poisoning
B. DDT poisoning
C. chronic lead poisoning
D. Thallium poisoning
E. salicylism

513. At age six months the normal infant

A. has good head control and sits with support
B. has developed good Moro reflex
C. has no Babinski sign
D. plays "peek-a-boo"
E. creeps well

514. At three months and in adults the following may be identical.
- **A.** Cerebrospinal fluid
- **B.** Electroencephalogram
- **C.** Nerve conduction velocity
- **D.** Percentage of time in REM sleep
- **E.** None of the above

515. A ten-year-old boy rapidly loses vision in both eyes. After a few weeks this becomes stationary. There are no other signs. A probable diagnosis is
- **A.** Friedreich's ataxia
- **B.** juvenile lipidosis (Kuf's)
- **C.** Leber's optic atrophy
- **D.** craniopharyngioma
- **E.** chromophobe adenoma

516. Peroneal muscular atrophy (Charcot-Marie Tooth) is
- **A.** usually transmitted as a dominant
- **B.** characterized by distal wasting in the hands and legs
- **C.** occasionally associated with Friedreich's ataxia
- **D.** compatible with normal life expectancy
- **E.** all of the above

517. A child repeatedly had painless injuries to the hands. One should suspect
- **A.** congenital indifference to pain
- **B.** familial dysautonomia
- **C.** syringomyelia
- **D.** none of the above
- **E.** all of the above

518. A nine-year-old child was mildly retarded, had swallowing difficulties, absence of tears, and unexplained episodes of hyperpyrexia. One could expect to find
- **A.** decreased tendon reflexes
- **B.** skin blotching
- **C.** convulsions
- **D.** postural hypotension
- **E.** any of the above

519. A child complains of low back pain radiating down one leg. There is also progressive urinary dysfunction and a tuft of hair is seen over the lumbar spine. One might suspect

- **A.** Klippel-Feil syndrome
- **B.** Arnold-Chiari malformation
- **C.** diastematomyelia
- **D.** spina bifida occulta
- **E.** none of the above

520. A common complication of acute purulent meningitis in children is

- **A.** endocarditis
- **B.** purulent arthritis
- **C.** subdural effusion
- **D.** paralytic ileus
- **E.** none of the above

DIRECTIONS: Each group of questions below consists of a list of lettered headings followed by a list of numbered words or statements. For **each** numbered word or statement, select the **one** lettered heading that is most closely associated with it. Each lettered heading may be selected once, more than once, or not at all.

Match the following useful diagnostic signs.

- **A.** Niemann-Pick disease
- **B.** Wilson's disease
- **C.** Von Hippel-Lindau
- **D.** Schilder's diffuse sclerosis
- **E.** Juvenile amaurotic

521. Kayser-Fleischer ring
522. Splenomegaly
523. Retinal pigmentation
524. Retinal angioma
525. Blindness

Match the following syndromes and their etiology.

A. ECHO
B. Coxsackie, Group A
C. Coxsackie, Group B
D. Mumps
E. Poliomyelitis

526. Herpangina, rash, encephalitis
527. Myalgia, pleurodynia, encephalitis
528. Parotitis, orchitis, encephalitis
529. Morbilliform rash and meningitis
530. Fever, diarrhea, paralysis

8 ADULT CLINICAL NEUROLOGY

DIRECTIONS: Each of the questions or incomplete statements below is followed by a list of suggested answers or completions. Select the **one** that is best in each case.

531. In Tangier disease
- **A.** low density lipoproteins are abnormally low
- **B.** serum cholesterol is increased
- **C.** splenomegaly is common
- **D.** pattern of inheritance is autosomal dominant
- **E.** none of the above

532. The fundoscopic finding of the "double-ring sign" indicates
- **A.** megalopapilla
- **B.** coloboma
- **C.** optic disc hypoplasia
- **D.** central retinal vein occlusion
- **E.** none of the above

533. Gaze-evoked nystagmus that increases with prolonged eccentric gaze is usually a sign of
- **A.** congenital nystagmus
- **B.** multiple sclerosis
- **C.** ocular myasthenia
- **D.** barbiturate intoxication
- **E.** none of the above

534. A 20-year-old man presents with one month of fevers, progressive confusion, headaches, and photophobia. Laboratory data include: ESR 9, CSF: 45 neutrophils, 50 lymphocytes, and 5 mononuclear cells/mm^3, glucose 52, protein 480. Opening pressure 300 mm. CT scan demonstrates ventricular enlargement. All blood, urine, CSF culture and serologies are negative. PPD is negative. EEG demonstrates high voltage delta over the right temporal region. Which of the following statements is true?

- **A.** This patient is likely to be suffering from Reye's syndrome
- **B.** The negative tuberculin test excludes the diagnosis of tuberculous meningitis
- **C.** The patient is likely to be suffering from Mollaret's meningitis
- **D.** This patient is likely to be suffering from tuberculous meningitis

535. The severely hypothermic patient

- **A.** should not lose consciousness until core body temperature falls below 32°C
- **B.** may develop ventricular arrhythmias at body temperatures between 32–34°C
- **C.** will demonstrate activity of low amplitude but normal frequency on EEG
- **D.** is frequently left with permanent neurologic deficit even when rapid rewarming techniques are applied
- **E.** none of the above

536. A patient presents with complaints of symmetrical distal dysesthesias and motor weakness involving all four limbs. General physical exam reveals transverse white lines in the nails.

- **A.** Nerve and muscle biopsy will be the procedure of greatest diagnostic value
- **B.** Heavy metal screen will be the test of greatest diagnostic value
- **C.** This patient probably suffers from the Bassen-Kornzweig syndrome
- **D.** This patient probably suffers from an inherited disease involving peripheral nerves
- **E.** None of the above

537. Diseases which predominantly involve small myelinated and unmyelinated fibers

- **A.** may produce a neuropathy characterized by selective loss of vibration and deep tendon reflexes
- **B.** may produce a neuropathy characterized by intact sensory action potentials
- **C.** include Fabry's disease, Riley-Day syndrome, and most toxic neuropathies
- **D.** none of the above
- **E.** A and B

538. Herpes zoster (shingles) is

- **A.** produced by the same virus as herpes simplex
- **B.** always sensory in its manifestations
- **C.** not related etiologically to varicella
- **D.** almost always confined to spinal nerves
- **E.** none of the above

539. Characteristics of Becker's muscular dystrophy include

- **A.** pattern of inheritance is autosomal recessive
- **B.** age of onset usually between age 10 and 25
- **C.** markedly elevated serum CPK activity
- **D.** cardiac involvement is common
- **E.** none of the above

540. The syndrome consisting of spontaneous crying, dysarthria, dysphagia, and hyperactive jaw jerk is called
- **A.** Wallenberg syndrome
- **B.** Weber syndrome
- **C.** pseudobulbar syndrome
- **D.** Millard-Gubler syndrome
- **E.** Benedikt's syndrome

541. A patient had a sudden onset of hemiplegia and contralateral ophthalmoplegia. The lesion is most likely in the
- **A.** frontal lobe
- **B.** lateral medulla
- **C.** mesencephalon
- **D.** pons
- **E.** paracentral lobule

542. Acute subdural hematoma is not easily differentiated from
- **A.** chronic subdural hematoma
- **B.** acute epidural hematoma
- **C.** cerebral thrombosis
- **D.** acute cerebral laceration
- **E.** subdural hygroma

543. Cataplexy is usually seen in
- **A.** grand mal epilepsy
- **B.** Kleine-Levin syndrome
- **C.** narcolepsy
- **D.** psychomotor epilepsy
- **E.** status epilepticus

544. A brother and sister in their twenties gave a history of blurred vision with no other complaints. Onset was sudden without progression or other symptoms. Vision was 20/200 bilaterally with pale discs and central scotomas. One should consider most likely
- **A.** familial multiple sclerosis
- **B.** Leber's optic atrophy
- **C.** hereditary optic atrophy
- **D.** chiasmatic arachnoiditis
- **E.** none of the above

545. Inflammatory occlusion of the retinal arteries occurs in
- **A.** periarteritis nodosa
- **B.** rheumatic fever
- **C.** giant cell arteritis
- **D.** systemic lupus erythematosus
- **E.** tuberculosis

546. The most common cause of cerebral thrombosis is
- **A.** hypertension
- **B.** arteriosclerosis
- **C.** diabetes
- **D.** syphilis
- **E.** collagen disease

547. A 32-year-old man had several erythematous macules and then developed anesthetic patches on the face and an ulnar neuropathy. One should suspect as most probable
- **A.** panarteritis nodosa
- **B.** lupus erythematosus
- **C.** leprosy
- **D.** diabetes
- **E.** Dejerine Sottas' disease

548. In Huntington's chorea
- **A.** dementia is a late development
- **B.** the average duration of disease is 10 years
- **C.** seizures occur
- **D.** men are more often affected than women
- **E.** none of the above

549. In the stage of spinal shock following traumatic transection of the spinal cord
- **A.** there are hyperactive deep reflexes
- **B.** there are absent deep reflexes
- **C.** there are absent superficial reflexes
- **D.** there is hypertonicity of the bladder
- **E.** there are absent deep and superficial reflexes

550. The following seizure does NOT occur following head injury.
A. Classic grand mal
B. Classic petit mal (absence)
C. Psychomotor
D. Focal motor
E. Jacksonian seizure

551. A 20-year-old man had a 10-year history of ataxia. On examination he had ataxia, loss of vibration and position sense nystagmus, absent deep reflexes in the legs, Babinskis, and club feet. The most likely diagnosis is
A. pseudosclerosis
B. multiple sclerosis
C. Marie's ataxia
D. Friedreich's ataxia
E. Refsum's syndrome

552. Clinical features of the Shy-Drager syndrome include all EXCEPT
A. orthostatic hypotension
B. anhidrosis
C. urinary incontinence
D. extrapyramidal symptoms
E. profound sensory disturbance

553. A 25-year-old woman complained of proximal weakness. This and proximal wasting were seen on examination. A muscle biopsy showed neurogenic atrophy. She most likely has
A. limb girdle dystrophy
B. hereditary amyotrophic lateral sclerosis
C. Wolfhart-Kugelberg-Wielander disease
D. Duchenne's dystrophy
E. polymyositis

554. In the differential diagnosis of spastic paraparesis of adult life, the condition that might be most easily excluded by neurological examination is
- **A.** hereditary amyotrophic lateral sclerosis
- **B.** syringomyelia
- **C.** familial spastic paraplegia
- **D.** cervical spondylosis
- **E.** multiple sclerosis

555. A syrinx most often occurs in the
- **A.** medulla
- **B.** cervical cord
- **C.** thoracic cord
- **D.** lumbar cord
- **E.** sacral cord

556. The diagnosis of syringomyelia depends primarily on the appearance of
- **A.** myelographic changes
- **B.** cerebrospinal fluid findings
- **C.** localized muscle atrophy, sensory changes, and dysmorphism
- **D.** electromyographic changes
- **E.** remissions in clinical course

DIRECTIONS: For each of the questions or incomplete statements below, **one or more** of the answers or completions given is correct. Select

- **(A)** if only 1, 2, and 3 are correct
- **(B)** if only 1 and 3 are correct
- **(C)** if only 2 and 4 are correct
- **(D)** if only 4 is correct
- **(E)** if all are correct

---

557. Down's syndrome is

1. more common among relatives of patients with Alzheimer's disease
2. associated with thyroid disease
3. associated with the neuropathologic changes characteristic of Alzheimer's disease
4. more common among relatives of patients with progressive dementias such as Pick's disease, Parkinson's disease, and Huntington's disease

A 40-year-old woman with rheumatoid arthritis has been managed with Ibuprofen 2400 mg/day, and D-penicillamine 500 mg/day for the past 5 years. She develops fluctuating ptosis, diplopia, and muscle weakness, all of which are exacerbated by repeated effort. Infusion of tensilon 5 mg rapidly reverses the neurologic symptoms. Several months after withdrawal of Ibuprofen and D-penicillamine, the symptoms resolve.

558. Which of the following statements is true?

1. This patient is likely to have elevated serum levels of antibody to acetylcholine receptor
2. This patient is likely to have an underlying thymoma, induced by immunosuppressive therapy
3. Treatment with anticholinesterase drugs is indicated during the symptomatic phase
4. This patient is likely to carry the HLA antigen DR4, but not A or B8

Directions Summarized

(A) 1, 2, 3 only; **(B)** 1, 3 only; **(C)** 2, 4 only; **(D)** 4 only; **(E)** all

559. Which of the following statements is true?
  1. This patient probably suffers from congenital myasthenic syndrome
  2. This patient could have myasthenia gravis, independent of her other immune mediated disease and treatment
  3. Ibuprofen is aggravating her underlying myasthenia gravis by producing postsynaptic receptor blockade
  4. D-penicillamine may be aggravating her underlying myasthenia gravis

560. Which of the following statements is true?
  1. This patient's symptoms might be worsened by treatment with corticosteroids
  2. This patient's symptoms are immune mediated and should be treated with high dose corticosteroids
  3. This patient may have thymic hyperplasia
  4. This patient should avoid nonsteroidal anti-inflammatory drugs in the future

561. In ophthalmoplegic migraine
  1. the ophthalmoplegia always occurs on the same side as the headache
  2. visual auras are unusual
  3. the headache may last several days
  4. it is more common in women

562. Adie's pupil
  1. may be bilateral
  2. may be associated with hypereflexia in the legs
  3. constricts with 1/8% pilocarpine
  4. is probably due to postganglionic sympathetic denervation of the ciliary muscle

563. Causes of pseudopapilledema include
1. drusen
2. hyaloid remnants
3. hyperopia
4. abnormal myelination of retinal nerve fibers

564. In true papilledema
1. SVP are always absent
2. there may be a familial etiology
3. visual acuity is usually diminished
4. the most specific ophthalmologic sign is opacification of the nerve fiber layer

565. A patient with thrombocytopenia, hypofibrinogenemia, and a prolonged prothrombin time
1. should be treated with corticosteroids if neurologic symptoms develop for small vessel vasculitis
2. may develop large vessel occlusion and stroke
3. may develop a diffuse encephalopathy from multiple small vessel occlusions, but should not develop large vessel occlusions
4. may develop subarachnoid hemorrhage

566. In Bell's palsy
1. hyperacusis develops in one-third of patients
2. taste is affected in one-third of patients
3. when hyperacusis develops, it signifies a lesion at, or proximal to, the temporal bone
4. when hyperacusis develops, it signifies a lesion distal to the chorda tympani

567. Sarcoid
1. involves the nervous system in 30% of patients
2. is associated with a lymphocytic, low glucose, CSF profile
3. is associated with a lymphocytic, normal glucose, CSF
4. involves the nervous system in 5% of patients

Directions Summarized

(A) 1, 2, 4 only; **(B)** 1, 3 only; **(C)** 2, 4 only; **(D)** 4 only; **(E)** all

---

568. Intracranial aneurysms definitely occur with increased frequency in patients with

1. fibromuscular dysplasia
2. polycystic renal disease
3. coarctation of the aorta
4. uncontrolled hypertension

569. Following rupture of an intracranial aneurysm, the probability of rebleeding is greatest

1. 30 days following the event
2. 20-30 days following the event
3. 30 days following the event, and stabilizes after the first year
4. 10 days and becomes stable 30 days after the event

570. The Vogt-Koyanagi-Harada syndrome is associated with

1. vitiligo, alopecia, and meningitis
2. sensorineural hearing loss
3. retinal detachments and papillitis
4. mental retardation and cardiac conduction abnormalities

571. Lacunar infarcts occur secondary to

1. lipohyalinosis
2. chronic meningitis
3. arterial dissection
4. valvular disease

572. The ataxia hemiparesis syndrome is
1. related to lacunar infarcts involving the corona radiata of the posterior limb of the internal capsule
2. related to lacunar infarcts involving the basis pontis
3. characterized by weakness of the leg with ipsilateral arm and leg ataxia
4. characterized by weakness of the leg and contralateral arm and leg ataxia

573. Refsum's disease
1. is due to an autosomal recessive inborn metabolic error
2. is characterized by phytanic acid accumulation
3. produces a chronic polyneuropathy, ataxia, and elevated CSF protein
4. has no known therapy

574. Fibromuscular dysplasia
1. may be associated with spontaneous arterial dissection
2. is more common in men than women
3. frequently involves bilateral carotid arteries
4. is one of the few indications for surgery for an "asymptomatic bruits"

575. A patient with hepatic porphyria develops seizures. Anticonvulsants which are relatively safe in this setting include
1. valproate
2. carbamazepine
3. phenytoin
4. paraldehyde

DIRECTIONS: Each group of questions below consists of a list of lettered headings followed by a list of numbered words or statements. For **each** numbered word or statement, select the **one** lettered heading that is most closely associated with it. Each lettered heading may be selected once, more than once, or not at all.

Match clinical findings with the appropriate structural level. Each structure may be used once, more than once, or not at all.

A. Forebrain
B. Midbrain
C. Pons
D. Medulla

576. Posthyperventilation apnea
577. Ataxic breathing
578. Apneustic breathing
579. Cheyne-Stokes respirations
580. Cluster breathing

A. Leptospirosis
B. Lyme disease
C. Syphilis
D. A, B, and C
E. None of the above

581. Illness caused by a spirochete
582. Aseptic meningitis, myositis, headache, fever, nephritis
583. Cryoglobulins detected in the serum
584. Illness caused by a rickettsia

Match the following.

- **A.** Bilateral optic neuritis and transverse myelitis
- **B.** Conglomerate translucent bodies of the nerve head
- **C.** Beri-beri optic neuritis
- **D.** Orogenital ulcers with chronic uveitis

585. Drusen
586. Devic's disease
587. Bechet's disease
588. Camp eye

Match the following tumors and description.

- **A.** Brainstem tumor
- **B.** Cerebellar hemispheric tumors (child)
- **C.** Fourth ventricular tumor
- **D.** Midline cerebellar tumor
- **E.** Commonest primary adult cerebellar tumor

589. Astrocytoma
590. Polar spongioblastoma
591. Hemangioblastoma
592. Medulloblastoma
593. Ependymoma

DIRECTIONS: Each set of lettered headings below is followed by a list of numbered words or phrases. For each numbered word or phrase select

(A) if the item is associated with A only
(B) if the item is associated with B only
(C) if the item is associated with both A and B
(D) if the item is associated with neither A nor B

A. Myasthenia gravis
B. Botulism
C. Both
D. Neither

594. Muscle weakness is the result of the inability of end plate potentials at a percentage of synapses to achieve threshold and trigger muscle action potentials
595. Prevents acetylcholine release from the presynaptic terminal
596. Characterized by marked facilitation
597. High frequency stimulation produces sequential decrement in the amplitude of the muscle action potential

DIRECTIONS: The group of questions below consists of a figure with lettered components, followed by a list of numbered words or statements. For **each** numbered word or statement the **one** figure or figure component that is most closely associated with it. Each figure or figure component may be selected once, more than once, or not at all.

Match Figures 8.1–8.3 with their corresponding descriptions.

A. Retinitis pigmentosa
B. Toxoplasmosis
C. Tigroid fundus
D. Hypertensive retinopathy

598. Figure 8.1
599. Figure 8.2
600. Figure 8.3

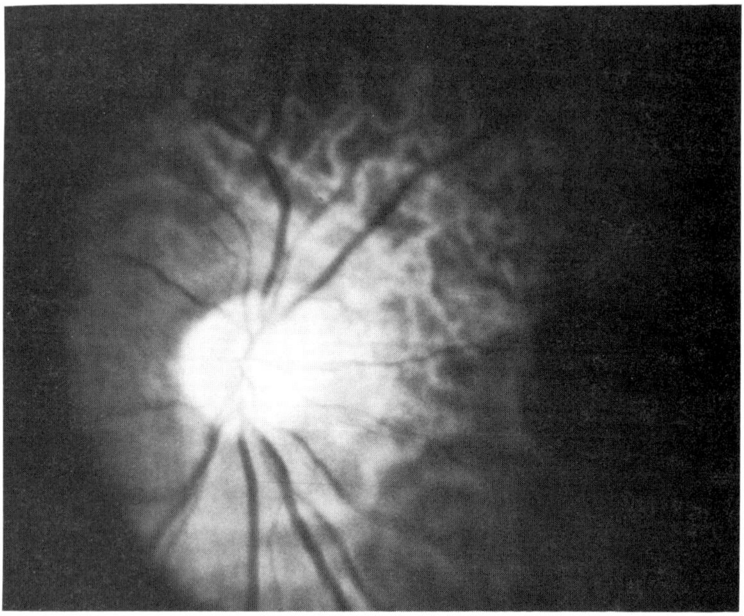

Figure 8.1

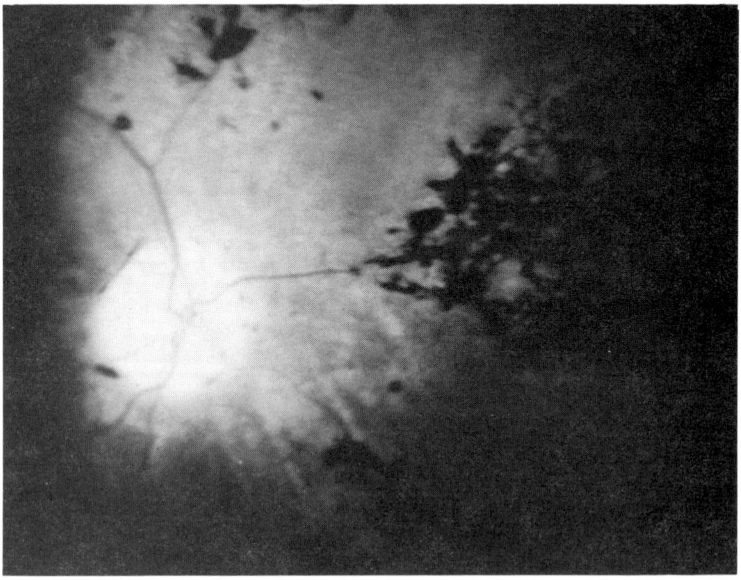

Figure 8.2

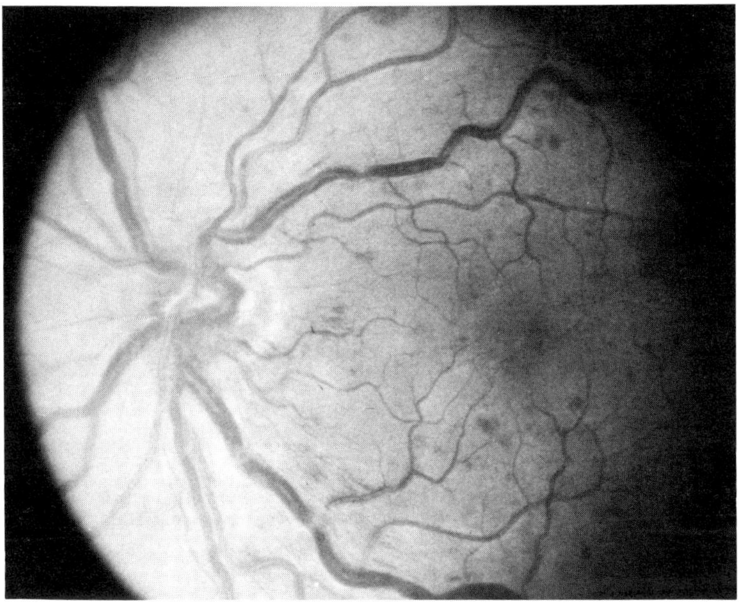

Figure 8.3

ANSWERS AND COMMENTS

The authors have made every effort to thoroughly verify the answers to the questions which appear on the preceding pages. However, as in any text, some inaccuracies and ambiguities may occur; therefore, if in doubt, please consult your references.

The Publisher

PART 1: NEUROANATOMY

1. **(A)** Internal arcuate fibers arise from the gracile and cuneate nuclei and form the medial lemniscus, which terminates in the VPL nucleus of the thalamus and carries kinesthetic sense and discriminative touch. **(REF:** 62, pp. 307-308**)**

2. **(C)** The lateral geniculate body is part of the visual system and receives the termination of the optic tract. **(REF:** 62, p. 473**)**

3. **(B)** The flocculus contains a group of Purkinje's cells that discharge in relation to the velocity of the eyes moving in space. Floccular lesions impair smooth visual tracking, and cause downbeat, gaze-evoked and rebound nystagmus, and postsaccadic drift. **(REF:** 54, pp. 916-917**)**

4. (C) The Lenticulostriate arteries supply the posterior portion of the anterior limb, the genu, and the anterior portion of the posterior limb of the internal capsule. **(REF:** 12, p. 558**)**

5. (C) The zone of Lissauer contains descending afferent fibers of the trigeminal nerve (in the medulla), which become the spinal trigeminal tract. The substantia gelatinosa becomes the spinal trigeminal nucleus. **(REF:** 62, pp. 301-302**)**

6. (B) The substantia gelatinosa primarily receives fibers of small dorsal root ganglion cells mediating pain and temperature, and may give rise directly to some fibers of the lateral spinothalamic tract. **(REF:** 12, p. 67**)**

7. (B) The ala cinerea is also called the trigonum vagi. The dorsal efferent nucleus of the vagus lies under it, along with the fasciculus solitarius. **(REF:** 12, p. 114**)**

8. (A) The ventricular fasciculus, or H2 bundle of Forel, arises from the globus pallidus. **(REF:** 12, p. 374**)**

9. (B) Fibers of the lateral lemniscus terminate in the inferior colliculus. The inferior colliculus in turn projects to the medial geniculate body. **(REF:** 12, p. 225**)**

10. (C) Corticobulbar fibers are carried in the genu of the internal capsule. **(REF:** 12, p. 396**)**

11. (B) The lateral lemniscus project to the medial geniculate nucleus of the thalamus via the inferior colliculus. **(REF:** 12, p. 273**)**

12. (B) Sensory impulses from the face project to the VPM nucleus of the thalamus. Sensory fibers for the rest of the body terminate primarily in the VPL nucleus. **(REF:** 12, p. 288**)**

13. (A) The fornicate lobe comprises the cingulate, isthmus, and hippocampal gyri, as well as the uncus. It is part of Broca's limbic lobe. **(REF:** 12, p. 249**)**

14. (B) The average weight of the male brain is about 1300 gm. The average female brain weighs about 1200 gm. **(REF:** 12, p. 410**)**

15. (B) Some fibers from the dentate nucleus bypass the red nucleus and pass directly to the VL nucleus of the thalamus. **(REF:** 12, p. 209**)**

16. (A) The major fascicles of the median olfactory area comprise the median forebrain bundle, which terminates premanil in the ventromedial hypothalamic nucleus. **(REF:** 12, p. 426**)**

17. (A) Pyramidal cells and layering are considered the hallmark of mature cortex. **(REF:** 12, p. 434**)**

18. (B) Lissauer's tract arises from the dorsal root ganglia and gives off collateral at all levels to the substantia gelatinosa. **(REF:** 12, p. 76**)**

19. (D) The medial striate or recurrent artery of Heubner arises from the anterior cerebral artery and supplies the lateral portion of the head of the caudate and contiguous portions of the putamen. **(REF:** 12, pp. 550–557**)**

20. (B) The thickness of average cortex is about 2.5 mm. Visual cortex ranges from 1.45 to 2.2 mm. **(REF:** 12, p. 410**)**

21. (B) The ventral or anterior spinocerebellar tract enters the cerebellum through the superior cerebellar peduncle. **(REF:** 62, p. 421**)**

22. (B) About 41% of total cortex is in the frontal lobe, 21% in the temporal lobe, and about 17% in the occipital lobe. **(REF:** 12, p. 410**)**

23. (B) Axons of the granule cells bifurcate in the molecular layer to form parallel fibers. **(REF:** 12, p. 195**)**

24. (D) Preganglionic sympathetic and parasympathetic fibers, and postganglionic parasympathetic fibers are cholinergic. Postganglionic sympathetic fibers to sweat glands are cholinergic. **(REF:** 12, p. 525**)**

25. (D) The spinotectal tract arises from the dorsal funicular grey matter, assumes a position on the medial border of the lateral spinothalamic tract, and eventually distributes to the superior colliculus. **(REF:** 12, p. 79**)**

26. (C) The ganglion cells of the retina give rise to optic nerve fibers. The ganglion cells receive impulses from the bipolar cells, which in turn receive impulses from light-stimulated rods and cones. **(REF:** 12, p. 277**)**

27. (B) The fastigial nucleus lies medial to the other deep cerebellar nuclei. The dentate nucleus is the most lateral. **(REF:** 12, p. 210**)**

28. (A) The Purkinje cells are the efferent neurons of cerebellar cortex. They project upon the deep cerebellar nuclei. **(REF:** 12, p. 193**)**

29. (A) The artery of charcot is a branch of the lenticulostriate arteries, which are derived from the middle cerebral arteries. **(REF:** 12, p. 558**)**

30. (C) Anterior thalamic and frontopontine radiations are carried in the anterior limb. Corticorubral fibers are contained in the posterior limb of the internal capsule. **(REF:** 12, pp. 396-397**)**

31. (A) Some of the visual projection fibers to the inferior calcarine cortex become Meyer's loop. **(REF:** 12, p. 457**)**

32. (B) Areas lacking the blood-brain barrier include the supraoptic crest, pineal gland, pituitary gland, area postrema, subfornical organ, and choroid plexus. The components of the blood-brain barrier are thought to include capillary endothelium, basement membrane, and astrocytic foot processes. The blood-brain barrier stains after injection of trypan blue, but filters the dye from surrounding neural tissues. The blood-brain barrier has been reported to be more permeable to basic (positively charged) dyes. **(REF:** 62, p. 224**)**

33. (D) The cuneocerebellar tract arises from cells of the accessory cuneate nucleus, which receives impulses from group Ia muscle fibers. This tract is the upper limb equivalent of the posterior spinocerebellar tract. **(REF:** 62, p. 273**)**

34. (D) The inferior cerebellar peduncle is also known as the restiform body. It contains primarily olivocerebellar fibers. Its tracts and fibers originate in the medulla and spinal cord. **(REF:** 62, p. 319**)**

35. (A) The dentate nucleus projects primarily to the ventral lateral nucleus of the thalamus. **(REF:** 62, p. 426**)**

36. (B)
37. (C)
38. (A)
39. (D) The anterior and posterior limbs of the internal capsule are supplied primarily by the striate branches of the middle cerebral artery. The thalamus is supplied by the thalamogeniculate and thalamoperforating branches of the posterior cerebral artery. The globus pallidus is supplied mostly by the anterior choroidal artery, which usually arises directly from the internal carotid. The anterior portion of the hypothalamus receives its blood supply from the anteromedian ganglionic branches of the anterior cerebral arteries. **(REF:** 672, pp. 70-27**)**

40. (C) Meissner's corpuscles are encapsulated receptors
41. (A) which are widely distributed in hairless skin and
42. (D) detect 2 point discrimination. The largest encap-
43. (B) sulated receptors, the Pacinian corpuscles, detect
44. (E) pressure and vibration. Merkel's discs are free nerve endings which are believed to be touch receptors that respond to deformation of the surface epidermis. Annulospiral afferents, or Ia afferents respond to muscle stretch. The Golgi tendon organs, or Ib afferents respond to stretch and muscle contraction. **(REF:** 62, pp. 76-88**)**

45. (B) The substantia gelatinosa is also known as lamina
46. (C) 2. Alpha motor neurons are contained in lamina IX.
47. (A) Renshaw cells are found in lamina VII. Cells of the
48. (D) nucleus proprius are found in lamina IV. **(REF:** 62, pp. 244-246**)**

49. (B) The fibers of the cochlear nerves originate in the
50. (A) spinal ganglia. Destruction of the cochlear nerves
51. (D) or both dorsal and ventral cochlear nuclei causes ipsilateral deafness. Since the secondary cochlear pathways are both crossed and uncrossed, lesions of one lateral lemniscus cause partial bilateral loss of hearing, most marked in the contralateral ear. The temporal lobe participates in sound localization. **(REF:** 62, p. 347**)**

52. (B) Lesions of the ventromedial hypothalamic nucleus
53. (C) produce hyperphagia. Lesions of the lateral hypo-
54. (A) thalamic nucleus impair the desire to feed. ADH
55. (E) secretion occurs mainly from the supraoptic nucleus. The paraventricular nucleus is responsible for secretion of oxytocin. **(REF:** 62, pp. 495-497**)**

56. (C) Horner's pupil results from interruption of the sym-
57. (B) pathetic pupillomotor pathways anywhere between
58. (A) the primary order neuron in the hypothalamus, the second order neuron in the cervicothoracic junction of the spinal cord, and the third order neuron in the superior cervical ganglion. Adie's pupil is thought to be due to short nerves to the ciliary muscle which then sprout into a denervated pupillary sphincter muscle, after injury to the ciliary

ganglion. The Argyll-Robertson pupils are thought to be due to disruption of central inhibitory pathways which disinhibit the Edinger-Westphal nucleus and result in hypertonicity of the pupillary sphincter. **(REF:** 54, pp. 866-877**)**

59. (D) This is the system of cytoarchitectural fields of
60. (A) the cortex according to Brodmann. **(REF:** 12, p.
61. (F) 440**)**
62. (B)
63. (G)
64. (C)
65. (E)

66. (C) VPM and VPL nuclei receive sensory information
67. (C) from the face and body and therefore project to
68. (A) somesthetic cortex. The medial geniculate body is
69. (B) part of the auditory pathway and projects to audi-
70. (D) tory cortex. The lateral geniculate body receives optic tract fibers and projects to visual cortex. The ventral tier nuclei receive input from many extrapyramidal systems and project to motor and supplementary motor cortex. **(REF:** 62, p. 464**)**

71. (B) The inferior cerebellar peduncle contains dorsal
72. (A) spinocerebellar tract, cerebellareticular fibers,
73. (A) vestibulocerebellar tract, dorsal and ventral super-
74. (C) ficial arcuate fibers cerebellospinal tract, arcuo-
75. (C) cerebellar fibers, vestibular or root fibers, olivo-
76. (A) cerebellar fibers, and trigeminocerebellar connec-
77. (C) tions. The superior cerebellar peduncle (brachium
78. (A) conjunctivum) contains cerebellotectal fibers,
79. (A) dentatorubral fibers, dentatothalamic fibers, cere-
80. (C) bellotegmental fibers, ventral spinocerebellar
81. (C) tract. The middle cerebellar peduncle (brachium pontis) carries pontocerebellar fibers. **(REF:** 12, pp. 200-207**)**

82. (B)
83. (B)
84. (A)
85. (C) The medial geniculate body receives fibers of the auditory pathway directly via the inferior colliculus. The lateral geniculate body receives the termination of the optic tract fibers. The medial longitudinal fasciculus contains both oculomotor and vestibular fibers and fibers of the reticular formation, which may contain auditory pathways which are involved in reflex closing of the eyes and turning the head in response to noise. **(REF:** 62, pp. 346, 353-354**)**

PART 2: NEUROPATHOLOGY

86. (C) Bunina bodies are irregularly shaped cytoplasmic inclusions seen in anterior horn cells of patients with ALS. **(REF:** 26, p. 310**)**

87. (B) A variant of Niemann-Pick disease, characterized by dementia, ataxia, and vertical ophthalmoplegia is associated with sea-blue histiocytes, found predominantly in bone marrow and lymph nodes. **(REF:** 42, p. 466**)**

88. (C) Marek's disease is a demyelinating peripheral neuropathy mediated by cellular immunity. The etiologic factor is a herpesvirus. **(REF:** 19, p. 46**)**

89. (B) Hunter-Russel syndrome is caused by methylmercury. Pathologically there is cerebellar and cerebrocortical atrophy. **(REF:** 30, pp. 546-547**)**

90. (C) The biochemical abnormality in Bassen-Kornzweig syndrome is absence of low density lipoproteins. There is extensive CNS and (to a lesser extent) peripheral demyelination. **(REF:** 42, p. 469**)**

91. (E) There are about 120 x 10^6 rods in the retina, and about 6-5 x 10^6 cones. Cone cells are receptors for color (photopic) vision. Light hyperpolarizes the cell membrane and inhibits release of neurotransmitter. Dopamine, glycine, taurine, and acetylcholine have all been identified in the retinal neurons. **(REF:** 53, p. 145**)**

92. (D) Polar spongioblastoma is a biologically and morphologically primitive tumor. It arises in the first or second decade near the third and fourth ventricles. It is locally invasive and may metastasize widely through the meninges. **(REF:** 47, p. 53**)**

93. (D) The pathological appearance is as described in parts A and B. The tumor may occur at any age but is most common in the fourth and fifth decades. **(REF:** 47, p. 85**)**

94. (A) Subependymal giant cell astrocytoma is a benign, slowly growing tumor which is characteristically associated with tuberous sclerosis. It tends to arise from the wall of the lateral ventricle and to gradually produce obstruction to CSF circulation. **(REF:** 47, pp. 40-41**)**

95. (D) Glioblastoma is more common in males. Medulloblastomas are more common in males. Astrocytomas affect men more than women. Intracranial schwannomas are more common in women, those in the spinal canal predominate in men. **(REF:** 47, pp. 55, 130, 206**)**

96. (B) The peripheral neuropathy of thiamine deficiency has segmental demyelination as a characteristic, but is also characterized by axonal degeneration as well. **(REF:** 22, p. 196**)**

97. (A) Hallervorden-Spatz disease usually presents in the first and second decades of life. Anterior horn cells are most affected. Changes in the cerebral cortex are not prominent. The basal ganglia give a strong iron-positive reaction due to increase of normal siderophilic pigment in these areas. **(REF:** 22, p. 178**)**

98. (C) Nissl substance is absent from the axon hillock. It is composed of rough endoplasmic reticulum. **(REF:** 22, p. 5**)**

99. (E) Cerebral lesions of toxoplasmosis often calcify. They may be present as large granulomatosis lesions, miliary lesions, or diffuse parenchymal inflammation with overlying meningeal inflammation. **(REF:** 22, p. 270**)**

100. (A) Carbon monoxide poisoning can also lead to sequelae of seizures, cortical blindness, and diffuse cognitive dysfunction. Pathologically, lesions are prominent in the globus pallidus. **(REF:** 22, pp. 68-69**)**

101. (C) The third, fifth, and sixth cortical layers are the most susceptible to hypoxia. Ammon's horn and the globus pallidus are most always involved in hypoxic lesions. Purkinje and basket cells of the cerebellum are the most vulnerable of cerebellar cortex cells to hypoxia. **(REF:** 22, p. 50**)**

102. (A) The primary lesions of lathyrism involve the pyramidal and spinocerebellar tracts and posterior columns. There may also be abnormalities of bone and cartilage. **(REF:** 22, p. 225**)**

103. (C) The medullary pyramids are rarely involved in SCSD. **(REF:** 22, p. 208**)**

104. (A) The Schwann cell is the myelin-forming cell of the peripheral nervous system. Central myelin is formed by the oligodendrocyte. **(REF:** 22, p. 30**)**

105. (C) Alzheimer's II glia are characteristic of Wilson's disease and have abnormally large nuclei with fine yellow brown granules in the nuclei. **(REF:** 22, p. 173**)**

106. (C) This is thought to happen when the temporal lobes are displaced through the incisura during birth. **(REF:** 22, p. 783**)**

107. (D) Lewy bodies are hyaline cytoplasmic inclusions characteristic of Parkinson's disease. **(REF:** 22, p. 612**)**

108. (A) After section of a nerve, the earliest changes are swelling of the axon, which may be seen after 12 hours. Next occurs disintegration of neurofibrils. Fragmentation of myelin is usually complete at the fourth day. **(REF:** 22, p. 697**)**

109. (E) Gitter cells are microglial cells that are transformed into so-called fatty macrophages. They first appear about 48 hours after tissue injury. **(REF:** 1, p. 173**)**

110. (C) Effects of cerebrovascular disease are seen in about 25% of all autopsy specimens (brains). However, it is the most common cause of nervous system disease. **(REF:** 1, p. 171**)**

111. (B) In purulent meningitis, subpial tissues are generally normal, but there may be foci of neurophilic leukocytic infiltrate, or cerebral infarction if venous occlusion occurs. **(REF:** 1, p. 106**)**

112. (A) Macrophages are recruited from blood vessels and appear first in perivascular tissues. **(REF:** 1, p. 86**)**

113. (A) Monocytes are more extensive in white matter than grey matter lesions. **(REF:** 1, p. 36**)**

114. (C) PTAH stains collagen. **(REF:** 1, p. 5**)**

115. (A) The neural plate, neural tube, and axial skeleton form during the third week and are derived from the notochord. **(REF:** 1, p. 331**)**

116. (A) Leakage of serum proteins into a subdural hematoma may be responsible for delayed swelling of the hematoma. **(REF:** 1, p. 225**)**

117. (C) It is unclear why posttraumatic epilepsy is not an immediate sequela of trauma. **(REF:** 1, p. 226**)**

118. (B) Patients with Wilson's disease have low serum ceruloplasmin. Spongy necrosis of the cortex and Alzheimer's type I glia occur but are uncommon. **REF:** 1, p. 250**)**

119. (B) SSPE is a leukoencephalopathy that is related to measles infection. **(REF:** 1, p. 137**)**

120. (B) Globoid bodies are a type of foreign body giant cell seen in Krabbe's leukoencephalopathy. **(REF:** 1, p. 284**)**

121. (C) Glioblastoma and metastatic tumors are the most common adult brain tumors. **(REF:** 1, pp. 304-305**)**

122. (A) Type A inclusion bodies are commonly seen in herpes encephalitis. **REF:** 1, p. 136**)**

123. (B) Hemangiomas are congenital arteriovenous malformations which may involve any part of the CNS. **(REF:** 1, p. 180**)**

124. (E) Neurofibrillary tangles are made up of neurofilament and neurotubules, and are seen in a variety of conditions. **(REF:** 26, p. 287**)**

125. (C) Hirano bodies are eosinophilic rodlike structures with a highly organized fine structure, that have been reported in several different neurological diseases. **(REF:** 26, pp. 291, 299**)**

126. (A) Wolman's disease is a rare condition characterized by absence of acid lipase and abnormal accumulation of cholesterol and triglycerides. **(REF:** 42, p. 468**)**

127. (D) The role of aluminum in the etiology and pathology of Alzheimer's disease has not yet been clearly elucidated. **(REF:** 26, p. 295**)**

128. (E) Benign intracranial hypertension may be caused in infants by vitamin A deficiency. **(REF:** 42, p. 504**)**

129. (E) Pathologically, muscle biopsies of patients with the Kearns-Sayre syndrome show ragged red fibers. **(REF:** 4, p. 405**)**

130. (A) The median eminence is part of the pituitary gland. **(REF:** 2, p. 346**)**

131. (D) Patients with Duchenne's muscular dystrophy,
132. (A) which is an x-linked recessive disorder, may de-
133. (C) velop contractures from very short periods of
134. (B) immobilization, or even muscle biopsy. Limb-girdle dystrophy is autosomal recessive and is characterized by early adult onset of proximal muscle weakness. Infants with nemaline myopathy, in addition to the characteristic facies, have congenital hypotonia with late motor milestones. Myotonic dystrophy is autosomal recessive with gonadal atrophy, frontal balding, and mental subnormality. **(REF:** 4, pp. 382, 393**)**

135. (C) Capillary hemangioblastomas are tumors of the
136. (A) posterior fossa which are classically associated
137. (A) with Von Hippel Lindau disease. They consist of
138. (A) hemangioblastomas of the CNS, angiomatosis of
139. (D) the retina, multiple renal and pancreatic cysts,
140. (B) and renal cell cancer. They are also associated
141. (C) with erythrocythemia, syringomyelia, and pheo-
142. (C) chromocytoma.

Capillary telangiectasias are malformations composed of capillaries separated by normal brain tissue. CNS lesions are rarely associated with Rendu-Osler-Weber disease. The most common site is the pons. Most are clinically silent.

Cavernous angiomas are also often clinically silent. They are associated with calcification and gliosis. They may occur in cortex, pons, and spinal cord. **(REF:** 47, pp. 235-245**)**

143. (B) Blepharoplasts are "aborted" cilia, found in ependymomas. **(REF:** 47, p. 107**)**

144. (D) The glioblastoma accounts for more than 50% of all gliomas. It is the most common primary brain tumor of adults. **(REF:** 47, p. 55**)**

145. (B)
146. (B) Ependymomas may arise in the hemispheres, adjacent to the third and fourth ventricles (particularly in the elderly), spinal cord (where they account for the majority of intramedullary spinal cord gliomas). Symptoms are caused by slowly evolving mass effect. **(REF:** 47, pp. 107-108**)**

147. (A)
148. (A) Medulloblastomas are malignant tumors of childhood which arise from the cerebellum. They are locally invasive, may spread through CSF pathways, and have been documented to metastasize to bone marrow. **(REF:** 47, p. 130**)**

149. (C) Psammoma bodies in meningiomas consist of calcium salts that have been laid down in degenerating tumor cells. **(REF:** 47, p. 177**)**

150. (A) See questions 147 and 148.

151. (E) Schwannoma, the most common primary spinal tumor, accounts for 29% of tumors within the spinal canal. **(REF:** 47, p. 206**)**

152. (E)
153. (E)
154. (B)
155. (C)
156. (D)
157. (B)
158. (A)
159. (E)
160. (C) Cysticercosis, the larval form of the pork tapeworm, taenia solium, produces cystic nodules throughout brain parenchyma. Meningoencephalitis and hydrocephalus may occur. Praziaquantel may be an effective treatment.

Echinococcus occasionally affects the brain. Hosts are dogs and sheep. In 2% of infected patients large cystic cystic brain lesions may be formed.

Toxoplasma gondii may be acquired by eating raw beef and contact with cat feces. Congenital infection may produce fever, rash, lymphadenopathy, cerebral calcification, microcephaly, and chorioretinitis. Acquired toxoplasmosis is strongly associated with immunosuppressed conditions, particularly AIDS. The brain in such cases shows large necrotic lesions with free and encysted T. Gondii. Large areas of necrosis may mimic mass lesions.

Cerebral amebiasis is caused by free-living flagellate amebas. The illness may begin with fever, gastroenteritis, and acute meningitis. Numerous cerebral microabscesses may be seen. Hepatitis is frequently associated with this condition. **(REF:** 39, pp. 1925-1931**)**

161. (F)
162. (A)
163. (D)
164. (E)
165. (C)
166. (B) All of these inborn errors of metabolism are leukodystrophies that are characterized by abnormal storage of various lipids and sphingolipids. The storage material that is accumulated depends on the particular biochemical defect. **(REF:** 1, pp. 284-286**)**

167. (B) Psammoma bodies are calcium deposits that are laid down in degenerating tumor cells. They are characteristic of meningiomas. **(REF:** 47, p. 177**)**

168. (H) Neurofibrillary tangles are characteristic of Alzheimer's disease. **(REF:** 22, p. 814**)**

169. (A) Unverricht's myoclonus is sometimes known as Lafora body epilepsy. These are cytoplasmic, concentric, rounded inclusions in the neuron. **(REF:** 22, p. 788**)**

170. (C) Antoni type A pattern of cells are compact bundles of thin, elongated cells that are strongly argyrophilic. They are common in acoustic neuromas. **(REF:** 47, p. 209**)**

171. (I) Lewy bodies are characteristic of Parkinson's disease. (See #107), **(REF:** 22, p. 612**)**

172. (G) Type A inclusions are intranuclear masses that are usually rounded with a clear halo. They are seen in various viral encephalitides. **(REF:** 22, p. 296**)**

173. (E) Rosenthal fibers are elongated, eosinophilic, degenerated glial cells seen in piloid astrocytomas. **(REF:** 47, p. 36**)**

174. (D) Opalski cells are large oval cells with small nuclei that are found primarily in the thalamus and basal ganglia of patients with Wilson's disease. **(REF:** 22, p. 174**)**

175. (F) Ependymomas classically contain rosettes, which are circles of glial cells around a central lumen. Pseudorosettes in ependymomas are perivascular, and the formations taper toward the blood vessel into a point. **(REF:** 47, p. 125**)**

PART 3: NEUROPHARMACOLOGY

176. (D) Amantadine releases dopamine from neuronal storage sites. **(REF:** 20, p. 238**)**

177. (B) Bromocriptine and Lisuride are ergot derivatives which act directly on dopamine receptors. Bromocriptine lowers G.H. levels in acromegaly and decreases the on-off phenomenon. **(REF:** 55, 949-956**)**

178. (D) Barbiturates and carbamazepine generally depress DPH levels. Sporadically, however, chloramphenical and phenobarbital may increase phenytoin levels. **(REF:** 46, pp. 2630-2631**)**

179. (A) Valproate is effective against absence, other spike and wave epilepsies, tonic clonic, and complex partial seizures. It elevates GABA concentrations in the brain by influencing the activity of GABA-transaminase. It interferes with the elimination of phenobarbital. **(REF:** 40, pp. 207-218**)**

180. (B) Although the incidence of birth defects may be multiplied by a factor of three in babies born to mothers taking phenytoin, the risks from seizures to mother and fetus outweigh the risk of teratogenicity. **(REF:** 40, pp. 207-218**)**

181. (E) Phenobarbital and phenytoin induce the metabolism of vitamin D in the liver, resulting in hypocalcemia and osteomalacia. **(REF:** 23, pp. 201-211**)**

182. (B) Pergolide is a long-acting postsynaptic dopamine which decreases parkinsonian symptoms. **(REF:** 25, pp. 509-513**)**

183. (C) The neuroleptic malignant syndrome occurs in the setting of phenothiazine use but is not dose related. The symptoms may be ameliorated by dopamine agonists. **(REF:** B, pp. 163-165**)**

184. (E) These are all side effects of bromocriptine. In addition hallucinations, confusion, and dyskinesias may be seen. **(REF:** 55, pp. 949-956**)**

185. (C) Ethambutal may produce optic neuritis, which is an indication to reduce the dosage. **(REF:** 57, p. 603**)**

186. (A) Isoniazid may produce a peripheral neuropathy in 17% of patients. This is due to pyridoxine (B-6) deficiency, which may also produce optic neuropathy or seizures. Isoniazid raises CNS GABA levels. **(REF:** 57, pp. 476-489**)**

187. (B) Tardive dyskinesias may remit spontaneously. They are best controlled with neuroleptic agents. Anticholinergic agents may aggravate the symptoms. **(REF:** 31, pp. 71-72**)**

188. (A) Bromocriptine may produce confusion and hallucinations. It is routinely used in doses in excess of 50 mg per day, and is a treatment for the on-off phenomenon. **(REF:** 31, pp. 63, 65**)**

189. (C) Propranolol may be used in doses greater than 240 mg for migraine treatment. A 6-month trial is warranted, as success may progressively increase during the first year. Relapse is common, and the dosage should be slowly tapered after control is achieved. **(REF:** 31, pp. 105-110**)**

190. (D) Neostigmine and edrophonium are anticholinesterases. A therapeutic trial may be of value diagnostically. Quinine and curare have been used in low doses or regionally to uncover latent myasthenia gravis. **(REF:** 20, p. 462**)**

191. (D) Atropine is an antimuscarinic anticholinergic agent. The autonomic ganglia and neuromuscular junction are nicotinic receptor sites. The parasympathetic neuroeffector junctions include salivary, bronchial, and sweat secretion. **(REF:** 20, p. 514**)**

192. (B) All of the agents are sympathetic effectors. Only norepinephrine, epinephrine, and isoproterenol have OH groups substituted on the 3 and 4 positions of the benzene ring, making them catecholamines. **(REF:** 20, p. 480**)**

193. (B) Opiates in a single therapeutic dose shift the EEG toward increased voltage and lower frequency such as occurs in natural sleep. **(REF:** 20, p. 250**)**

194. (B) Atropine methylnitrate is a quartenary ammonium compound with poor CNS penetration. D-tubocurarine works primarily at the neuromuscular junction. Hexamethonium works at the level of the autonomic ganglion. Physostigmine is an anticholinesterase. Scopolamine is an antimuscarinic with CNS action. **(REF:** 20, pp. 514-525**)**

195. (B)
196. (A) Tyramine is the active substance. It is present in aged cheeses and, to a lesser extent, in beer, red wine, chicken liver, yeast, and pickled herring. **(REF:** 20, p. 183**)**

197. (B) The autonomic nervous system consists of two efferent divisions, the sympathetic or thoracolumbar outflow, and the parasympathetic or craniosacral outflow. **(REF:** 14, p. 405**)**

198. (A) Atropine and D-tubocurarine produce competitive blockade of acetylcholine receptors while decamethonium and succinylcholine are depolarizing blocking agents. **(REF:** 20, p. 579**)**

199. (E) Transmission from motoneuron collaterals to the Renshaw cells (interneurons which are inhibitory to motoneurons of the same segmental level) is cholinergic. The receptors are nicotinic. **(REF:** 16, p. 62**)**

200. (B) Hemicholinium blocks the transport system which allows choline to accumulate in nerve terminals, and therefore blocks ACh synthesis. **(REF:** 20, p. 434**)**

201. (D) The transmitter of all preganglionic autonomic fibers and all postganglionic parasympathetic fibers is ACh. **(REF:** 20, p. 404**)**

202. (D) Pilocarpine acts postsynaptically, primarily at muscarinic receptors. **(REF:** 20, p. 472**)**

203. (C) Nausea results from stimulation of the chemoreceptor trigger zone for emesis, located in the area postrema of the medulla. **(REF:** 20, p. 251**)**

204. (E) Hemicholinium interferes with the ACh synthesis and therefore has an anticholinergic effect. **(REF:** 20, p. 433**)**

205. (B) Norepinephrine is the precursor of epinephrine. **(REF:** 20, p. 423**)**

206. (C) The enzyme is L-aromatic amino acid decarboxylase, which converts dopa to dopamine. **(REF:** 20, p. 423**)**

207. (B) Tyrosine hydroxylase is the rate limiting enzyme. It converts tyrosine to L-dopa. **(REF:** 20, p. 423**)**

208. (C) There is no evidence that antihistamines are of use in treating tertiary syphilis. Antihistamines have anticholinergic properties that may relieve some extrapyramidal symptoms. **(REF:** 20, pp. 610, 611**)**

209. (A) In man 5-HT undergoes oxidative deamination by monamine oxidase to form 5 hydroxyindoleacetic acid. **(REF:** 20, p. 621**)**

210. (D) The effects of D-tubocurarine begin to fade within 20 minutes of the initial dose due to redistribution of the drug. **(REF:** 20, p. 585**)**

211. (C) Zarontin (ethosuximide) is the agent of choice for petit mal epilepsy. **(REF:** 20, p. 212**)**

212. (E) See Question 201.

213. (D) Edrophonium is a reversible carbamate inhibitor belonging to the same class of drugs as physostigmine. **(REF:** 20, p. 450**)**

214. (E) See Question 190. Hexamethonium is a ganglionic blocker. Quinine, like curare, decreases the excitability of the motor end plate, so that responses to acetylcholine are reduced. **(REF:** 20, p. 1063**)**

215. (D) Guanethidine is the only agent listed which does not induce liver G-ALA synthetase activity and is safe to use in the setting of acute intermittent porphyria. **(REF:** 49, p. 309**)**

216. (D)
217. (A)
218. (C)
219. (B) Norepinephrine is the direct precursor of epinephrine, but as dopamine is the precursor of norepinephrine, it is also a precursor of epinephrine. Norepinephrine is contained in postganglionic symptatotic fibers. Epinephrine is localized in adrenal chromaffin cells. Studies of spinal motoneurons reveal a cholinergic pathway. **(REF:** 49, pp. 404, 421, 423**)**

220. (A) Paroxysmal hemicrania best responds to treatment with indomethacin. **(REF:** 21, pp. 159-163**)**

221. (B) Lithium is an effective prophylactic treatment for cluster headache. **(REF:** 21, pp. 159-164**)**

222. (C) Prednisone is a treatment for acute cluster headache. **(REF:** 21, pp. 159-163**)**

223. (E) Inderal may intensify vascular headaches by displacing serotonin from platelets. **(REF:** 54, p. 986**)**

224. (C) REM sleep appears to be initiated by firing of cholinergic neurons in the pons. Muscarinic agonists will mimic this action and reduce REM latency. Serotonin synthesis inhibitors do not reduce REM latency. Tricyclic antidepressants suppress REM sleep. REM latency is consistently decreased in primary affective disorders. **(REF:** 64, p. 889**)**

225. (C) Seizures generally are not a manifestation of opiate withdrawal. Excessive sweating and "gooseflesh" rather than dry skin is seen. **(REF:** 20, p. 296**)**

226. (E) The fever produced by hypothalamic injection of prostaglandin is dose dependent and not affected by aspirinlike drugs. It also produces marked sedation, potentiates the effect of barbiturates, and gives some seizure protection against electroshock. **(REF:** 53, pp. 321, 322**)**

227. (B) GABA and glycine are excluded from brain. **(REF:** 53, pp. 321, 322**)**

228. (A) So far there has not been demonstrated a link between adenylate cyclase and substance P. **(REF:** 53, p. 299**)**

229. (E) The neurologic complications of fluorosis are generally a result of bone distortions, exophytic growth, and brittle bones, which occur from excess deposition of fluoride. **(REF:** 30, p. 527**)**

230. (E) Naloxone, an opiate antagonist, has been shown to reverse actions of different analgesics. **(REF:** 53, p. 265**)**

231. (B) Ethosuximide is the drug of choice for petit mal seizures, although indications are that valproate may be as effective. Valproate is more effective than ethosuximide in the treatment of tonic clonic seizures. At present valproate is used as adjuvant therapy (with DPH or carbamazepine) in the treatment of complex partial seizures. Valproate shows promise as a treatment for atonic seizures. **(REF:** 7, pp. 661-666**)**

232. (A) The side effects of valproate include sedation, nausea, hair loss, bleeding tendencies, hepatic toxicity, weight gain, and tremor. **(REF:** 7, pp. 661-666**)**

233. (B) Barbiturate metabolism is interfered with by valproate. Valproate's effect on phenytoin is less consistent and rarely necessitates a change in dosage. **(REF:** 7, pp. 661-666**)**

234. (A) Quinidine, aminoglycosides, and tetracyclines all have mild neuromuscular blocking effects. **(REF:** 5, pp. 409-413**)**

235. (C) Phenytoin and chlorpromazine interfere with presynaptic calcium ion influxes. **(REF:** 5, pp. 409-413**)**

236. (B) Benzodiazepines are effective in the treatment of status epilepticus. Their effect on spinal reflexes is primarily central, residing in the brainstem reticular system. Benzodiazepines bind more frequently in the cerebellum than in the spinal cord. **(REF:** 34, p. 618**)**

237. (A) Baclofen and dantrolene sodium are effective in patients with spinal cord transection. Dantrolene treats spasticity by interfering with excitation-contraction coupling, by decreasing the release of Ca^{++} from sarcoplasmic reticulum. **(REF:** 34, p. 618**)**

238. (E) All of these agents have been reported to produce dystonia. **(REF:** 3, p. 124**)**

239. (D) Propranolol is an effective treatment for benign essential tremor but apparently renders its effect through central mechanisms. Therefore, sufficient time must elapse for the drug to penetrate the blood-brain barrier before tremor control is achieved. **(REF:** 3, pp. 126, 127**)**

240. (D) Aspirin is a potent inhibitor of cyclooxygonase, which is a key enzyme in the conversion of arachidonic acid into prostaglandin. The inhibitory action appears to be due to irreversible acetylation of cyclooxygenase. **(REFS:** 18 and 53, p. 314.

PART 4: NEUROPHYSIOLOGY

241. (E) The neuronal NA^+/k^+ pump is coupled to an ATP which is located in the cell surface membrane. It is activated by external K^+ and internal Na^+. The rate of Na^+ extrusion from the cell is unaltered by changes in resting potential, although it is quite sensitive to the concentration of Na^+ ions inside the cell. **(REF:** 28, pp. 66-67**)**

242. (D) Increased permeability to K^+ hyperpolarizes the cell, producing an inhibitory effect. **(REF:** 53, pp. 173-174**)**

243. (A) Secretion and exocytosis of synaptic vesicles appear to be regulated by influx and efflex of calcium. **(REF:** 53, p. 207**)**

244. (B) Release of GABA on to the presynaptic terminal causes increased permeability to CI^- and CI^--dependent depolarization in the presynaptic terminal. **(REF:** 53, p. 174**)**

245. (C) Lesions of the hippocampus, fornix, and mamillary bodies produce severe short-term memory deficits such as those seen in patients with Korsakoff's syndrome. **(REF:** 62, p. 537**)**

246. (C) The intensity/frequency relationship of receptors depends on the rate of depolarization. **(REF:** 48, p. 144, Vol. IV**)**

247. (B) The lateral hypothalamus appears to be a hunger center. Lesions produce aphagia and adipsia. **(REF:** 48, p. 658, Vol. I**)**

248. (B) After increased permeability to Na^+ that occurs after the action potential, there is persistent increased permeability to K^+ which causes hyperpolarization of the membrane as it returns to the K^+ equilibrium potential. **(REF:** 48, pp. 284-285, Vol. IV**)**

249. (B) The resting membrane potential is -70 mv. The equilibrium potential for Na^+ is +60 mv. **(REF:** 48, p. 285, Vol. IV**)**

250. (C) Inhibitory impulses increase permeability to K^+ and cCl^- and drive the membrane potential toward -80mv, the mean of the CI^- and K^+ equilibrium potentials. **(REF:** 48, p. 291, Vol. IV**)**

251. (D) The larger the Na^+ current, the steeper is the rate of rise of the action potential. Also, the higher the concentration of highly mobile ions, the greater the current flow. **(REF:** 48, pp. 88-89, Vol. IV**)**

252. (D) Gradation of contractile force of a muscle is accomplished by recruitment of additional motor units and repetitive discharge in individual motor units. **(REF:** 48, p. 172, Vol. IV**)**

253. (D) Local anesthetics block nerve conduction in any type of nerve fiber. Therefore, if they do not block large myelinated fibers, they will block smaller efferents. **(REF:** 20, p. 379**)**

254. (C) Failure to recognize the names of body parts is generally associated with dominant hemisphere lesions. All other symptoms listed may be referable to the nondominant hemisphere (hemineglect, visuospatial apraxia). **(REF:** 37, p. 577**)**

255. (B) Slow muscle fibers are also called "red" muscle. **(REF:** 48, p. 210, Vol. IV**)**

256. (B) At high rates of firing, the postsynaptic neuron may not respond to each of a series of presynaptic impulses because of the obligatory refractory period that follows each action potential. **(REF:** 48, p. 262, Vol. IV**)**

257. (D) Stimulation of the otoliths by linear acceleration or tilt produces compensatory eye movements that tend to stabilize the eyes. Counterrolling refers to conjugate compensatory torsional movement of the eyes during lateral tilt. **(REF:** 27, p. 716**)**

258. (C) The alpha component is produced by the rapid conduction myelinated A fibers; the beta component is produced by slower conducting myelinated B fibers. Because conduction velocity is different, separation increases at sites more distant from stimulating electrodes. **(REF:** 48, p. 76**)**

259. (D) The motor unit is the functional unit of contraction. **(REF:** 48, p. 171, Vol. IV**)**

260. (A) A group Ia afferent volley discharges homonymous motoneurons but enhances the excitability of heteronymous synergistic muscles. **(REF:** 48, pp. 276-277, Vol. IV**)**

261. (C) It is thought that the mechanism of presynaptic inhibition is to limit the amount of neurotransmitter released from activated excitatory knobs. **(REF:** 48, p. 297, Vol. IV**)**

262. (B) The chemical quanta producing the MEPP is pocket of neurotransmitter contained in synaptic vesicles. **(REF:** 27, pp. 1333-1334**)**

263. (D) The Kluver-Bucy syndrome includes loss of fear and aggression. **(REF:** 48, pp. 674-675, Vol. I**)**

264. (A) The earliest reflexes to return after spinal shock are withdrawal reflexes. **(REF:** 48, p. 2, Vol. I**)**

265. (C) Stimulation of the inhibitory reticular formation inhibits the patellar response, reduces decerebrate rigidity, and decreases movement in response to stimulating the motor cortex. **(REF:** 48, p. 17, Vol. I**)**

266. (D) There are no direct connections between the olfactory tract fibers and the thalamus. However, the prepyriform cortex does project to the dorsomedial thalamic nuclei. **(REF:** 48, p. 335, Vol. I**)**

267. (A) The currently held view is that the cerebral cortex functions in terms of gross movement, not individual muscles, and there is multiple representation of muscle groups for different movements. **(REF:** 48, p. 77, Vol. I**)**

268. (B) The overall ratio is two thin filaments for every thick filament. **(REF:** 48, p. 177, Vol. IV**)**

269. (A) Frequency is affected by resistance and impedance properties of a system, which in the ear is affected by the elastic and mass properties of the bony conduction system. **(REF:** 48, p. 364, Vol. I**)**

270. (D) Electrical stimulation of the thalamocortical system evokes slow waves over a large part of the cerebral hemispheres. Repetitive stimulation produces incremental increase in amplitude (recruiting; augmenting). This phenomenon is not observed with sensory stimulation distal to the thalamus. **(REF:** 37, p. 256**)**

271. (C) Granule cells are types of neurons found in the cerebellum. **(REF:** 48, p. 472, Vol. I**)**

272. (C) The receptive fields of retinal ganglion cells have an annula organization in which the center and periphery are mutually antagonistic. **(REF:** 48, p. 489, Vol. I**)**

273. (D) The cortical cell is most sensitive to contours (e.g., edges and lines) and the spatial orientation of these contours. **(REF:** 48, p. 531, Vol. I**)**

274. (D) The olivocochlear bundle (bundle of Rasmussen) is a major inhibitory pathway of impulses leaving the cochlea. **(REF:** 48, pp. 394-395, Vol. I**)**

275. (A) Tetraethylammonium acts on the potassium channel. **(REF:** 53, p. 103**)**

276. (D) The ventromedial nucleus is a satiety center. **(REF:** 48, p. 657**)**

277. (J) The lateral hypothalamus is a feeding center. **(REF:** 48, p. 657**)**

278. (I) The lateral geniculate nucleus receives retinal impulses through the optic tracts. **(REF:** 48, p. 517**)**

279. (B) Stimulation of the thalamic relay nucleus produces a cortical response which grows rapidly in amplitude. This is known as the augmenting phenomenon. **(REF:** 37, p. 259**)**

280. (E) The C.M. thalamic nucleus is one of the nuclei within the generalized thalamocortical system within which electrical stimuli will evoke recruiting responses in cerebral cortex. **(REF:** 37, p. 256**)**

281. (F) The cingulate gyrus is part of the limbic system, which has major influences on emotion and behavior. **(REF:** 62, pp. 538-539**)**

282. (A) The septal nuclei contain cholinergic neurons, which reportedly produce pleasurable sensations when stimulated. **(REF:** 48, p. 680, Vol. I**)**

283. (H) All cerebellar cortical output is inhibitory whether it goes to deep nuclei or to the vestibular complex. **(REF:** 37, p. 731**)**

284. (G) The mesencephalic reticular formation is reciprocally connected with the hypothalamus, septum, basal ganglion, and preoptic region. High frequency electrical stimulation of this area produces EEG activation arousal. **(REF:** 37, pp. 266-267**)**

285. (C) The reticulospinal neurons reside in the pons and medulla. Stimulation produces inhibition of spinal reflexes. **(REF:** 37, p. 265**)**

PART 5: NEUROCHEMISTRY

286. (C) Uptake of choline into the cell is the rate-limiting step for acetylcholine synthesis. **(REF:** 53, p. 191**)**

287. (B) The cell bodies of beta-endorphinergic neurons are located in the arcuate nucleus of the hypothalamus, and their nerve tracts project into the periacqueductal grey. **(REF:** 53, p. 202**)**

288. (C) A glycoprotein, pro-opiocortin is presumed to be the precursor to ACTH and beta-lipotropin. The sequences of beta-endorphin and melanocyte-stimulating hormone are contained in beta-lipotropin. **(REF:** 53, p. 263**)**

289. (C) The brain consumption of oxygen is about 49 ml of O_2/min, or about 20% of resting total body oxygen consumption. **(REF:** 2, p. 305**)**

290. (D) Mannose crosses the blood-brain barrier and is converted to mannose-6-phosphate, and then fructose-6-phosphate, replacing glucose in the glycolytic pathway. **(REF:** 2, p. 311**)**

291. (D) Brain phosphofructokinase is inhibited by ATP. **(REF:** 2, p. 173**)**

292. (C) A ganglioside is a sphingoglycolipid that contains sialic acid. **(REF:** 2, p. 210**)**

293. **(C)** Patients with Leigh's disease, or subacute necrotizing encephalomyelopathy, are not able to synthesize thiamine triphosphate. **(REF:** 53, p. 666**)**

294. **(D)** Sphingomyelin is a relatively minor component of myelin. Lecithin is a major component. The major lipid components are as listed. **(REF:** 2, p. 378**)**

295. **(D)** The major mechanism for terminating the actions of catecholamines is reuptake into nerve terminals. The uptake process is energy dependent and is linked to sodium uptake. **(REF:** 53, p. 2009**)**

296. **(B)** LSD-25 contains an indole 6 structure, which makes it resemble serotonin. **(REF:** 2, p. 600**)**

297. **(E)** Triglycerides and free fatty acids are only found in very small amounts in the brain. Brain lipids are almost all composed of cholesterol, phospholipid, and glycolipid. **(REF:** 2, p. 218**)**

298. **(D)** Patients with McArdle's disease have a defect in muscle phosphorylase and are unable to fully utilize glycogen in the glycolytic pathway. **(REF:** 53, p. 553**)**

299. **(B)** Cerebral O_2 consumption falls when blood glucose is reduced to an average of 19 mg dl. **(REF:** 2, p. 310**)**

300. **(C)** The brain is almost exclusively restricted to glucose as its m ajor oxidizable fuel. **(REF:** 2, p. 308**)**

301. **(B)** Infusion of dopamine into the third ventricle causes increased plasma FSH and LH, and decreased plasma prolactin. **(REF:** 2, p. 348**)**

302. **(E)** All of these substances have been demonstrated to act as neurotransmitters or neuromodulators in the CNS. **(REF:** 53, p. 162**)**

303. (B) The criteria needed to categorize a substance as a neurotransmitter are as follows: 1) the transmitter is present in nerve terminals; 2) the transmitter is released from nerve stimulation; 3) the postsynaptic effects of the neurotransmitter are the same as those caused by stimulation of the presynaptic nerve; 4) the dose-response curve of the putative neurotransmitter is altered by drugs in the same manner as are the natural synpatic potentials; 5) a mechanism exists locally to inactivate the transmitter. **(REF:** 53, p. 163**)**

304. (D) Malignant hyperpyrexia is a genetically determined susceptibility to certain anesthetics. It is fatal if untreated. The defect seems to be an abnormality of calcium metabolism in the muscle. Muscle biopsies from patients with the disease show abnormally strong contracture when exposed to caffeine. **(REF:** 4, p. 409**)**

305. (A) Cell bodies of dopaminergic neurons are located primarily in the midbrain, and have nigrostriatal, mesocortical, and tuberohyrophysical projections. Septo-hippocarpal pathways are primarily cholinergic. **(REF:** 53, p. 211**)**

306. (B) Monoamine oxiclose degrades norepinephrine. The major metabolite of norepinephrine in the periphery is VMA. The major metabolite in the brain is MHPG. **(REF:** 2, p. 92**)**

307. (A) The action of acetylcholine is terminated by acetylcholinesterase. **(REF:** 2, p. 100**)**

308. (D) Some GABA receptors are coupled to the benzodiazapine recognition site. **(REF:** 53, p. 236**)**

309. (A) Glutamate and aspartate are powerful cxcitatory
310 . (B) neurotransmitters. GABA and glycine hyperpo-
311. (A) larize the neuronal membrane and are major in-
312. (B) hibitory transmitters. **(REF:** 53, pp. 256-284**)**

313. (A) Tay-Sachs disease, or GM2 gangliosidosis, is characterized by a defect of hexogamidase A and an accumulation of monosialoceramdetrihexose. **(REF:** 42, p. 458**)**

314. (D) Gaucher's disease is a defect in glucocerebrosidase and an abnormal accumulation of glucocerebroside. **(REF:** 42, p. 462**)**

315. (C) The cherry-red spot results from deposition of neuronal storage material in the peripheral macula, which renders it pale and accentuates the red center. It is seen in several neuronal storage diseases. **(REF:** 42, p. 418**)**

316. (C) Five clinical variants of both Tay-Sach's and Niemann-Pick disease are recognized. **(REF:** 42, pp. 459, 465**)**

317. (B) Niemann-Pick disease is characterized by abnormal accumulation of sphingomyelin. **(REF:** 42, p. 465**)**

318. (A) Sandhoff's disease is an infantile variant of GM2 gangliosidosis. **(REF:** 42, p. 458**)**

319. (A) Type A Niemann-Pick disease presents in infants with hepatosplenomegaly and failure to thrive. **(REF:** 42, p. 465**)**

320. (B) Krabbe's disease and metochromatic leukodystro-
321. (A) phy are both leukoencephalopathies that can also
322. (C) involve the peripheral nervous system. The stor-
323. (C) age product in Krabbe's disease is galactocerebroside; the storage material in metachromatic leukodystrophy is cerebroside sulfate. **(REF:** 42, pp. 463-464**)**

324. (B) The endogenous opiates, endorphins and enkepha-
325. (A) lins, differ in their distribution and types of anal-
326. (B) gesia produced. The enkephalins inhibit the re-
327. (B) lease of substance P in the spinal cord. Analgesia
328. (C) produced by B-endorphin lasts several hours.
329. (D) **(REF:** 53, pp. 261-264, 290**)**

330. (C) The cell bodies of B-endorphin containing neurons are located in the arcuate nucleus of the hypothalamus. **(REF:** 53, p. 262**)**

331. (A)
332. (D) The supraoptic nucleus is primarily involved with vasopressin secretion; oxytocin is secreted by the paraventricular nucleus, although there is some crossover. **(REF:** 2, p. 344**)**

333. (B) Cell bodies containing substance P are located in periaqueductal grey, spinal and cranial sensory ganglia, basal ganglia, and the nucleus of the spinal trigeminal tract. **(REF:** 53, p. 279**)**

334. (A)
335. (C)
336. (D) Myosin is found in the A band and contains ATPase. Thin filaments made of actin are found in the I band. Tropomyosin is found in thin filaments and confers Ca^{++} dependence on the contractile system. Tropomyosin is strategically located between actin and myosin, so that in the absence of Ca^{++}, the ATPase activity of myosin is inhibited. **(REFS:** 2, p. 388; 48, p. 181, Vol. IV**)**

337. (C) Carbon tetrachloride can produce optic atrophy and encephalopathy. **(REFS:** 50, p. 88; 57, p. 616**)**

338. (A) Manganese intoxication produces damage to the substantia nigra, globus pallidus, and other extrapyramidal structures, and results in clinical manifestations similar to Parkinson's disease. **(REF:** 57, p. 619**)**

339. (B) Lead neuropathy is characteristically an axonal degeneration. It affects the upper limbs before the lower limbs in adults, and characteristically presents with wrist drop. **(REF:** 57, p. 496**)**

340. (E) The characteristic signs of organic mercury poisoning are paresthesias, visual disturbances, and ataxia. **(REF:** 57, p. 513**)**

341. (B) Botulinum toxin acts on the neuromuscular junction by binding to a high affinity site on the presynaptic membrane and inhibiting acetylcholine release. **(REF:** 53, p. 514**)**

342. (C) Alpha bungarotoxin initially binds to the presynaptic nerve terminals and increases acetylcholine release; later acetylcholine release is decreased. It also acts postsynaptically and binds irreversibly to cholinergic receptors. **(REF:** 53, p. 514**)**

343. (A) Black widow spider venom binds to the presynaptic membrane and alters calcium channels, causing massive release of acetylcholine. **(REF:** 53, p. 518**)**

344. (C) Vitamin B_{12} deficiency can produce diffuse demyelination in spinal cord, optic nerves, cerebral white matter, and peripheral nerves. **(REF:** 53, p. 669**)**

345. (A) Niacin deficiency results in central chromatolysis, with degeneration of Betz cells in the motor cortex. **(REF:** 53, p. 672**)**

346. (D) Paresthesias and "burning feet" are seen in patients deficient in pantothenic acid. Lesions of peripheral nerves are seen. **(REF:** 53, p. 673**)**

347. (B) Pyridoxine deficiency has been reported to lower seizure threshold, particularly in children. Pyridoxine-dependent enzymes act as catalysts for many metabolic pathways involving amino acids, glycogen, and unsaturated fatty acids. **(REF:** 53, p. 666**)**

348. (A)
349. (B)
350. (C) Exocytosis has been shown to be calcium dependent in all systems in which it occurs. Neurons are high in intracellular K^{++}; increased permeability to Na^+ and efflux of K^+ depolarizes, or excites, the neuron. **(REF:** 53, pp. 161, 173**)**

PART 6: DIAGNOSTIC NEUROLOGY

351. (C) Tenting of the dura usually indicates an acute or subacute condition. In a chronic condition, the dura becomes elongated and no longer produces a tentlike deformity. **(REF:** 60, p. 1218**)**

352. (C) The middle meningeal artery is usually a branch of the maxillary artery, which is itself a branch of the external carotid artery. The intracranial tumor that is most likely to have contributing blood supply from the external carotid artery is a meningioma. **(REFS:** 60, p. 751; 62, p. 79**)**

353. (D) Optic gliomas are usually slow growing and produce enlargement rather than atrophy of the optic canal. They produce a flattening of the sella tyrcica. Radiologic appearance of a "double" optic foramen is produced by the optic canal and the caroticoclinoid foramen. **(REF:** 60, pp. 105-108**)**

354. (C) Lead poisoning in children can produce increased intracranial pressure and widening of cranial sutures. Chronic exposure also produces increased density at the ends of rapidly growing long bones. **(REF:** 60, pp. 154-158**)**

355. (C) The most common of the pituitary adenomas which cause sella enlargement are the chromophobe adenomas. **(REF:** 60, p. 79**)**

356. (B) The presence of irritability in a paralyzed muscle after 2-3 weeks is a good prognostic sign. Initially, there may be no EMG evidence of motor unit activity on effort. **(REF:** 6, p. 557**)**

357. (C) Glomus jugulare tumors are highly vascular masses that characteristically produce bone destruction in the region of the jugular foramen. **(REF:** 60, p. 127**)**

358. (C) In clinical measurements of NCV, the ratio of the distance between the two points of stimulation and the time difference gives the conduction velocity of the fastest motor fiber in the nerve between the two points being studied. **(REF:** 6, p. 579**)**

359. (B) Meningiomas may have thousands of small calcifications that appear cloudlike on x-ray. **(REF:** 60, p. 194**)**

360. (D) Meningiomas commonly produce hyperostosis, increased vascular markings of the skull, and contain calcification, sometimes called psammoma bodies. **(REF:** 60, p. 194**)**

361. (E) Meningioma of the optic canal and ophthalmic artery aneurysm may produce enlargement of the optic foramen with erosion. Neurofibromatosis and optic nerve glioma may produce enlargement without erosion. **(REF:** 60, pp. 106–108**)**

362. (C) Cerebellopontine angle masses usually produce posterior and upward displacement of AICA, elevation of the superior cerebellar artery, lateral and backward displacement of the basilar artery, and compression of the petrosal vein. **(REF:** 60, p. 826**)**

363. (C) This is the most important angiographic sign of anterior hippocampal herniation. **(REF:** 60, p. 661**)**

364. (B) The sphenoid wings are commonly so defectively formed in patients with neurofibromatosis that they appear absent in a frontal projection in skull films. **(REF:** 60, p. 157**)**

365. (E) All of these conditions here have been associated with cerebral arteritis, which can produce arterial narrowing (spasm), aneurysm, or arterial occlusion. **(REF:** 60, pp. 1034-1037**)**

366. (C) Calcification is less common in chromophobe adenomas. **(REF:** 60, p. 196**)**

367. (B) Spondylolisthesis usually results from congenital malformations of the vertebral arch, or disease, e.g., degenerative, of the apophyseal joints. **(REF:** 60, p. 1157**)**

368. (C) Oligodendrogliomas are the leading cause of gliomatous calcification because they are more common tumors. **(REF:** 60, p. 211**)**

369. (A) Barbiturates cause widespread fast activity, maximally in the central and frontal regions. **(REF:** 60, p. 428**)**

370. (B) Intracranial calcifications in CMV may be stippled, nodular, or curvilinear. It is characteristically periventricular. Toxoplasmosis may produce calcification periventricularly or in the basal ganglia. The cysticercus embryo may become calcified in brain tissue. The calcification in tuberous sclerosis is estimated to occur in about 50% of cases. **(REF:** 60, pp. 219-229**)**

371. (E) K complexes are a bi- or triphasic wave followed by a sleep spindle. They are components of normal sleep. **(REF:** 56, p. 203**)**

372. (C) In lesions of fibrous dysplasia, there may be areas of increased density within the radiolucent area. **(REF:** 60, p. 119**)**

373. (D) Early after occurrence of a subdural hematoma, CSF shows gross blood and increased protein and the fluid becomes xanthochromic with increased protein and increased pressure. Slightly xanthochromic fluid with increased pressure and moderately increased protein is very characteristic of a developing subdural hematoma. **(REF:** 13, p. 789**)**

374. (B) Most patients above 40 years of age, especially women, exhibit calcium loss and osteoporosis. **(REF:** 60, p. 151**)**

375. (B) Types of gliomas which may be found intraventricularly include gangliogliomas, ependymomas, oligodendrogliomas, and astrocytomas. **(REF:** 60, pp. 427-430**)**

376. (A) Tumors in parietal, temporal, or occipital lobes do not produce this change in the anterior cerebral artery. **(REF:** 60, p. 670**)**

377. (D) Independent multifocal spikes may be seen in partial simple seizures, partial complex seizures, or generalized seizures. **(REF:** 56, p. 310**)**

378. (B) The H reflex is a monosynaptic reflex. It is an indicator of proximal nerve dysfunction. It is generated with subthreshold stimuli, it is blocked at supramaximal stimuli. It appears before the M response. **(REF:** 50, p. 230**)**

379. (A) Degeneration of sensory fibers accompanies postganglionic lesions such as plexopathies. Preganglionic lesions such as root avulsion or syringomyelia preclude regeneration of sensory fibers. **(REF:** 29, pp. 415-429**)**

380. (A) Temporal dispersion occurs because impulses of slow-conducting fibers lag increasingly behind those of fast-conducting fibers over a long conduction path. This produces an action potential of greater duration and smaller amplitude. Temporal dispersion alters sensory nerve potentials more than compound muscle action potentials. **(REF:** 29, pp. 415-429**)**

381. (A) Stimulation of the supraorbital nerve elicits a reflex response of the orbicularis oculi. This reflex response, as well as measurement of distal facial nerve excitability, is most often normal in trigeminal neuralgia. **(REF:** 29, pp. 415-429**)**

382. (B) Submaximal stimulation best elicits the electrically elicited stretch reflex, or H reflex, by stimulating Ia sensory afferent fibers. **(REF:** 29, pp. 415-429**)**

383. (E) Nerve conduction velocity is faster in proximal segments, between the ages of 5 years and 40 years, in shorter individuals, and at warmer limb temperatures. **(REF:** 29, pp. 415-429**)**

384. (A) Iophendylate (Pantopaque) myelography produces subclinical arachnoiditis in up to 67% of patients. Clinical symptoms are rarer and generally appear within months following myelography. **(REF:** 27, pp. 469-484**)**

385. (A) Metrizamide produces acute rather than chronic reactions. Adhesive arachnoiditis is rare. Metrizamide is less dense than CSF, so that positioning will not completely eliminate dye entry into the intracranial cavity. **(REF:** 27, pp. 469-484**)**

386. (B) See Question 383. Although nerve conduction velocity declines with age, the decrease is less than 10 m/sec by the sixtieth to eightieth year. Velocity decreases by about 2.4 m/sec/degree as temperature near the nerve falls from 38° to 29°C. **(REF:** 29, pp. 415-429**)**

387. (C) Although seizures and brain edema may complicate arteriography, they are rarer than indicated in choices A and B. **(REF:** 27, pp. 469-484**)**

388. (D) Spinal seizures following IV contrast dye administration are a rare complication, but have been reported in association with spinal cord AVM. **(REF:** 27, pp. 469-484**)**

389. (C) CSF pleocytosis is the most common complication of iophendylate myelography. See Question 384 for a discussion of adhesive arachnoiditis. **(REF:** 27, pp. 469-484**)**

390. (B) VER abnormalities in Parkinson's disease are presumably due to dopaminergic deficiency, based on confirmatory animal studies. **(REF:** 38, pp. 484-490**)**

391. (E) Brainstem auditory evoked responses have been reported to be abnormal in 21-55% of patients with MS with no clinical evidence of brainstem involvement. High doses of barbiturate do not alter the BAER. Comatose patients who have no more IV or V have been shown in one study to be less likely to survive. **(REF:** 9, pp. 1146-1147**)**

392. (B) The Martin-Gruber anomaly is a communication from the median to the ulnar nerve at the level of the forearm. It occurs in 15-20% of the population. **(REF:** 29, pp. 418-419**)**

393. (A) Bilateral synchronous rhythmic delta activity is a more common abnormality in older persons than younger ones. **(REF:** 56, p. 217**)**

394. (E) Increased beta activity may be seen in all of these conditions, as well as hyperthyroidism, early hepatic coma, and metachromatic leukodystrophy. **(REF:** 56, pp. 428-429**)**

395. (D) Hyperventilation responses are more common in younger persons. They normally end one minute after HV ceases and may include bursts and runs of synchronous delta activity. They are enhanced in hypoglycemia or cerebral anoxia. **(REF:** 56, pp. 221-222**)**

396. (A) See Question 390. **(REF:** 38, p. 65**)**

397. (B) See Question 390. **(REF:** 38, p. 65**)**

398. (A) After the fifth decade VER latency increases by
399. (B) approximately 2 m/sec per decade. Decreasing
400. (C) body temperature causes small changes in BAER
401. (C) interpeak latencies. Women have shorter P 100 and interpeak latencies than men, possibly related to brain and head size. All three types of evoked potentials are useful in indicating subclinical abnormalities. **(REF:** 9, pp. 1141, 1145**)**

402. (A)
403. (E)
404. (A)
405. (E) In neuroapraxia, conduction ceases without structural changes in the axon. Demyelination may occur. In axonotmesis there is loss of axonal continuity and Wallerian degeneration. In neurotmesis there is complete separation of nerve and Wallerian degeneration. Four to five days following nerve injury, stimulation distal to the lesion gives rise to no action potential, if Wallerian degeneration occurs. **(REF:** 29, p. 413**)**

406. (B)
407. (C)
408. (A)
409. (D) Stage 1 is a transitional stage with mixed frequency, low-voltage theta activity. Sleep spindles, 12-15 mz cycles appear in stage 2. Delta activity appears in stages 3 and 4. Sawtooth waves of 3-5 mz are present during REM sleep. **(REF:** 63, p. 87a**)**

410. (D)
411. (A)
412. (B, C)
413. (C)
414. (E) The EEG of patients with Jakob-Creutzfeld disease is often characterized by periodic sharp or periodic slow waves. Triphosic waves are usually seen in metabolic encephalopathies; they may be seen in postanoxic encephalopathy. Burst suppression is seen in severe cases of cerebral depression, usually anoxic encephalopathy, hypothermia, CNS depressant drugs. K-complexes are normal patterns of sleep. **(REF:** 56, p. 319**)**

415. (B) Intramedullary tumors expand the spinal cord and decrease the space between the spinal cord and the dye column. **(REF:** 60, p. 1172**)**

416. (C) Extramedullary, intradural tumors always displace the spinal cord and produce a well-delineated defect in the dye column. **(REF:** 60, p. 1194**)**

417. (A) Extradural tumors may compress the dural sac and collapse the subarachnoid space so that the dye column tapers to a point. **(REF:** 60, p. 1201**)**

418. (E) This condition occurs most often in women; it stops before reaching the midlife. **(REF:** 60, p. 9**)**

419. (C) This condition is also known as osteopetrosis. **(REF:** 60, p. 8**)**

420. (A) Usually the arches as well as the bodies of the fused vertebrae are joined in Klippel-Feil. **(REF:** 60, p. 1155**)**

421. (B) This condition is also associated with hypotelorism. **(REF:** 60, p. 50**)**

422. (D) In a platybasia skull, the angle obtained by tracing a line from the nasion to the tuberculum sella, and from there to the anterior margin of the foramen magnum, measures more than 143°. **(REF:** 60, p. 51**)**

423. (B) In Dandy-Walker syndrome, the cerebellum is malformed and the foramena of Luschka and Magerdie are atretic. **(REF:** 60, pp. 848-849**)**

424. (D) Luckenshadel is thought to be due to a disturbance in ossification, and may sometimes be a result of increased intracranial pressure in utero. **(REF:** 60, p. 64**)**

425. (A) This condition has no clinical significance. **(REF:** 60, p. 65**)**

426. (C) This is usually found in association with increased intracranial pressure. **(REF:** 60, p. 139**)**

427. (B) This is also called dolichocephalic cranistenosis. **(REF:** 60, p. 46**)**

428. (E) This is also called brachycephalic craniostosis. **(REF:** 60, p. 46**)**

429. (A) These are the characteristic radiographic findings of Crouzon's disease. **(REF:** 60, p. 47**)**

430. (C) There is associated elevation of the superior lateral aspect of the orbit and depression of the floor of the middle fossa and the petrous pyramid. **(REF:** 60, p. 49**)**

431. (D) There is usually premature closure of the coronal suture and finger abnormalities such as syndactylism. **(REF:** 60, p. 53**)**

432. (C) The width of the increased curvature of the thalamostriate vein is proportional to the degree of ventricular dilatation. **(REF:** 60, p. 727**)**

433. (D) This is characteristic of cerebellopontine masses. **(REF:** 60, p. 826**)**

434. (B) Characteristic of anterior temporal masses, also characteristic of elevation of the horizontal position of the middle cerebral artery. **(REF:** 60, p. 704**)**

435. (A) This finding is the most characteristic angiographic sign of a subfrontal mass. **(REF:** 60, p. 676**)**

436. (B) The beaded vessels are thought to represent immature vessels and sinusoids. Drainage of deep veins is usually an indication of a malignant intracerebellar growth. **(REF:** 60, p. 764**)**

437. (A or D) Characteristic of meningioma but may also be seen in other vascular neoplasms. The sunburst probably is due to a radial distribution of the small arterial branches which arise from the original site of the tumor blood supply. **(REF:** 60, p. 752**)**

438. (A or D) Characteristic of meningiomas. **(REF:** 60, p. 756**)**

439. (C) Metastatic tumors are usually fed by a single artery, which is usually not the case with glioblastoma. **(REF:** 60, p. 765**)**

440. (C) Characteristic of frontal (presylvian) masses. **(REF:** 60, p. 670**)**

441. (A) Seen with parasagittal masses, although the normal pericollosal artery may appear somewhat depressed. **(REF:** 60, p. 691**)**

442. (B) The most characteristic and most common finding with infrasylvian tumors. **(REF:** 60, p. 699**)**

443. (D) Forward displacement of the sylvian point is the most important finding in retrosylvian tumors. The angiographic sylvian point is usually found where the last branches of the middle cerebral artery emerge onto the surface of the brain. **(REF:** 60, p. 711**)**

444. (E) Displacement of the internal cerebral vein almost always occurs with thalamic tumors. **(REF:** 60, p. 719**)**

445. (C) Metastatic lesions of the skull are usually purely destructive and involve the outer and inner table. The outlines may be ragged and irregular. **(REF:** 60, p. 120**)**

446. (B) Pacchonian granulations result from projections of arachnoid granulation. They produce depressions on the inner tables of the skull. They are usually 2-3 cm from the midline. **(REF:** 60, p. 6**)**

447. (A) Venous lakes are present entirely within the diploë and do not involve the inner and outer table. Veins can be traced into most of them. **(REF:** 60, p. 120**)**

448. (D) As explained in Ref. 58, the labeled wave forms
449. (B) correspond to the anatomic correlates.
450. (E)
451. (A)
452. (C)

453. (E) The CT demonstrates an enhancing lesion in the thalamus, most compatible with a thalamic glioma. No other diagnostic choice should exhibit a focal thalamic lesion. **(REF:** 8, p. 695**)**

454. (D) The NMR demonstrates increased signal emanating from periventricular and discrete regions in white matter. The lesions are diffusely distributed, without mass effect or vascular pattern. This is most compatible with multiple sclerosis. **(REF:** 8, pp. 759-777**)**

455. (J) The ventricles are dilated. There is smooth periventricular increased signal, possibly representing increased subependymal water content. This is most compatible with a diagnosis of NPH. **(REF:** 8, pp. 686-688**)**

456. (B) There is an area of increased signal intensity in the pineal region, most compatible with a diagnosis of pineal tumor. **(REF:** 8, p. 695**)**

457. (F) There is a right temporal lesion of mixed signal intensity with mass effect. It does not follow a vascular distribution. The area of increased signal probably represents edema. This is most compatible with a diagnosis of astrocytoma. **(REF:** 8, p. 695**)**

458. (H) This is an NMR on a patient with no neurologic disease. **(REF:** 8, p. 854**)**

459. (G) In contrast to Question 458, there is pontine and cerebellar atrophy. This patient suffers from OPCA. **(REF:** 8, p. 651**)**

460. (A) There is an area of low density without mass effect extending in the distribution of the (L) MCA. This is most compatible with a (L) MCA infarct. **(REF:** 8, p. 655**)**

461. (I) The basal ganglia exhibit markedly increased signal intensity (compare the appearance with Question 465). This patient has Wilson's disease. **(REF:** 60, p. 606**)**

462. (C) This is a frontal carotid angiogram. **(REF:** 60,
463. (D) pp. 576-592**)**
464. (E)
465. (B)
466. (A)

467. (F) This is an NMR of a normal subject. The shadows
468. (G) are labeled with anatomic correlates. **(REF:** 60,
469. (C) p. 606**)**
470. (E)
471. (D)
472. (I)
473. (A)
474. (B)
475. (H)

PART 7: PEDIATRIC NEUROLOGY

476. (A) A 3-year-old child can stand on one foot, although he confuses the right and left foot. Plantar responses become flexor in 100% of normal children at age 2. Tonic neck reflexes are lost in early infancy. Opticokinetic nystagmus can be easily elicited from about 6 weeks of age. **(REF:** 17, pp. 11-13**)**

477. (B) The biochemical basis of metachromatic leukodystrophy is a deficiency of the enzyme arylsulfatase A. This deficiency permits the abnormal accumulation of sulfatide in tissues, which react with certain dyes, to produce metachromasia in the tissues that are stained. **(REF:** 17, pp. 350-351**)**

478. (A) Children with phenylketonuria classically have dry skin and hypopigmentation of hair and eyes; 25% of patients have eczema. Mental retardation may be minimized if dietary intake of phenylalamine is restricted from birth, or shortly thereafter. **(REf;** 17, pp. 300-301**)**

479. (E) The most common agent causing bacterial meningitis in children 6 months to 4 years of age is *H. influenza.* Most meningitides occurring during the first year of life are due to *E. coli* and the group B-beta hemolytic streptococci. **(REF:** 17, pp. 460-461**)**

480. (C) Most meningitis cases following head trauma occur 2 weeks postinjury. **(REF:** 17, p. 461**)**

481. (E) Meningitides in newborns are most likely to be due to *E. coli* and group B-beta hemolytic streptococci. **(REF:** 17, p. 460**)**

482. (B) Clear cerebrospinal fluid is more commonly associated with viral or leptrospiral meningitides. **(REF:** 17, p. 459**)**

483. (E) Acute purulent meningitis commonly shows several hundred to several thousand polymorphonuclear cells, increased protein, and markedly decreased sugar. **(REF:** 17, p. 459**)**

484. (C) CSF in tuberculous meningitis usually shows opalescent or clear fluid with less than 500 leukocytes/ml, which are predominantly mononuclear cells. Sugar content is decreased. **(REF:** 17, p. 459**)**

485. (D) Partially treated purulent meningitis may produce cerebrospinal fluid with moderate numbers of leukocytes which may be up to 50% mononuclear cells, with slightly decreased sugar content and elevated protein. **(REF:** 17, p. 465**)**

486. (B) Children with a brain abscess may have clear or opalescent CSF, usually under elevated pressure. The cellular reaction in a majority of cases is mononuclear. Protein varies from 50 mg% to 200 mg%. **(REF:** 17, p. 481**)**

487. (C) The CSF profile in tuberculosis meningitis, i.e., mononuclear and polymorphonuclear pleocytosis with modestly decreased sugar, may be similar to that seen in partially treated bacterial meningitis. **(REF:** 17, p. 465**)**

488. (E) Acute bacterial meningitis usually produces a predominantly polymorphonuclear pleocytosis. **(REF:** 17, p. 459**)**

489. (C) Focal cerebral infections may arise either by direct invasion through the skull or hematogenous spread of infection from an extracranial site. **(REF:** 17, pp. 475, 476**)**

490. (C) Occlusion of the ophthalmic veins produces exophthalmos and chemosis. The third, fourth, sixth, and first two divisions of the fifth cranial nerve pass through the cavernous sinus. **(REF:** 17, pp. 485-486**)**

491. (D) This picture may also be seen with subdural empyema. **(REF:** 17, p. 482**)**

492. (B) Among the more common subtertorial childhood tumors are cerebellar astrocytoma, medulloblastoma, and brain stem glioma. **(REF:** 17, p. 519**)**

493. (A) Abducens nerve palsy is a common, nonlocalizing sign of increased intracranial pressure. **(REF:** 17, p. 552**)**

494. (C) Vomiting secondary to increased intracranial pressure is common in children with posterior fossa tumors. **(REF:** 17, p. 551**)**

495. (D) Morning headache is particularly common in children with subtentorial tumors. **(REF:** 17, p. 551**)**

496. (B) Craniopharyngioma are more common in children. **(REF:** 17, p. 558**)**

497. (B) These signs are characteristic of cerebellar lesions. **(REF:** 17, p. 552**)**

498. (C) These signs tend to occur more commonly with cerebellar astrocytoma than with more malignant cerebellar tumors. **(REF:** 17, p. 555**)**

499. (D) Recurrences of medulloblastoma may also occur within the ventricular system. **(REF:** 17, pp. 556-557**)**

500. (A) All of the other tumors are more common in children than adults. **(REF:** 17, p. 549**)**

501. (A) The median age of diagnosis of optic nerve glioma is 7 years of age. Diagnosis may be accomplished by orbital tomography. **(REF:** 17, p. 562**)**

502. (C) The arteriovenous malformation of the vein of galen in the newborn produces massive shunting of blood into the venous circulation. **(REF:** 17, p. 590**)**

503. (B) Trauma is the most common cause of childhood intracranial hemorrhage, but hemorrhage may also be seen in children with AVM, aneurysm, blood dyscrasias, hypertension, intracranial neoplasm, hepatic disease, or vitamin deficiency. **(REF:** 17, p. 586**)**

504. (C) Fat embolism is usually associated with long bone fractures, and reach the brain via the pulmonary circulation and the left side of the heart. **(REF:** 17, p. 583**)**

505. (D) Clinical manifestation of cerebral AVM most commonly occurs during late childhood, adolescence, or young adulthood. **(REF:** 17, p. 591**)**

506. (A) Along with the conjunctival telangiectasia, pathologic findings include degeneration of the cerebellum and abnormalities of the thymus and lymphoid tissue. Differential diagnosis includes Arnold Chiari malformation and other cerebellar disorders associated with metabolic defects. **(REF:** 17, p. 620**)**

507. (E) These are characteristic features of Bassen-Kornzweig syndrome (abetalipoproteinemia). **(REF:** 17, p. 680**)**

508. (A) These are also features of Bassen-Kornzweig syndrome. Other somatic abnormalities include low hairline, webbed neck, and small external ears. **(REF:** 17, p. 624**)**

509. (B) This is also known as Dejerine-Sottas disease or hereditary motor sensory neuropathy type III. Other symptoms may include ataxia, nystagmus, and aberrant pupillary responses. **(REF:** 17, p. 675**)**

510. (C) Pathology of the CNS in thallium intoxication shows engorgement of cortical blood vessels with those neurons of the pyramidal tracts, globus pallidus, and substantion nigra being particularly affected. Peripheral neuropathology reveals a "dying-back" axonal degeneration. **(REF:** 17, p. 427**)**

511. (C) Etiology of familial spastic paraplegia is not known. It usually presents with stiffness and weakness in the legs during childhood or early adult life. **(REF:** 17, p. 656**)**

512. (C) These are characteristic signs of lead poisoning. **(REF:** 17, pp. 421-423**)**

513. (A) The Moro reflex is usually suppressed by age 4 months. Plantar responses remain extensor until 1-2 years of age. Babies play "peek-a-boo" at about 10 to 11 months of age and creep at about 10 to 11 months of age. **(REF:** 17, pp. 12-13**)**

514. (A) Nerve conduction velocities may be slower than normal adults in children less than 3 years of age. EEGs change as the central nervous system matures. Cerebrospinal fluid value may be close to that of an adult at 3 months of age. Newborns and young infants spend more time in REM sleep than adults. **(REF:** 17, pp. 35-41**)**

515. (C) Leber's optic atrophy is sex-linked and occurs six times more frequently in males than females. There is selective degeneration of the papulomocular bundle of the optic nerve, and primary neuronal degeneration of the retina. **(REF:** 17, p. 635**)**

516. (E) The differential diagnosis of Charcot-Marie-Tooth includes environmental intoxications and other hereditary neuropathies. **(REF:** 17, p. 673**)**

517. (E) All of these conditions may produce sensory loss in the upper extremities. **(REF:** 17, p. 677**)**

518. (E) These are features of familial dysautonomia, or Riley-Day syndrome. **(REF:** 17, p. 677**)**

519. (C) These are characteristic signs of diastematomyelia. The spinal cord is divided into two parts by a fibrous septum, usually in the low thoracic or lumbar region. Diagnosis may be made by netizamide computed tomography. **(REF:** 17, p. 651**)**

520. (C) Subdural effusion as a complication of purulent meningitis may be bilateral or unilateral and should be suspected in patients with unsatisfactory response after 72 hours of antibiotic treatment. **(REF:** 17, p. 463**)**

521. (B) This results from deposition of pigment in the cornea. **(REF:** 17, p. 612**)**

522. (A) Splenomegaly occurs due to abnormal storage of sphingomyelin. **(REF:** 17, p. 353**)**

523. (E) The "cherry-red" macula seen in Tay-Sach's disease results from loss of cells from the macula, with exposure of the vasculature of the choroid. Pigmentary retinal degeneration is also seen in some of the hereditary ataxias and diseases of metabolic defects such as Refsum's syndrome. **(REF:** 17, pp. 110-111, 349**)**

524. (C) Patients with von-Hippel-Lindau disease may have multiple hemangiomas in the central nervous system. **(REF:** 17, p. 57**)**

525. (D) This is also called spongy degeneration of the nervous system. Symptoms include failure to thrive, progressive paralysis, optic atrophy and ultimate blindness, and arrest of mental development. **(REF:** 17, p. 112**)**

526. (B) These viruses usually affect children age 5 to 9 years and are most prevalent in the summer months. Meningitis may occur with either type A or B infections. **(REF:** 17, p. 491**)**

527. (C) See Question 526.

528. (D) Inflammatory reaction to mumps virus may also occur in the pancreas, ovaries, or breast. **(REF:** 17, p. 493**)**

529. (A) Echo virus infections usually occur in the summer and fall. The aseptic meningitis may occur with or without skin rash. **(REF:** 17, p. 492**)**

530. (E) Poliovirus resides in the human gastrointestinal tract and can produce meningitis and paralysis after hematogenous spread to the central nervous system occurs. **(REF:** 17, p. 487**)**

PART 8: ADULT CLINICAL NEUROLOGY

531. (C) Tangier disease is a disorder characterized by absence of serum high density lipoproteins, a low serum cholesterol, and massive deposition of cholesterol within organs and tissues. It is autosomal recessive. **(REF:** 50, p. 93**)**

532. (C) The "double ring" is produced by the outline of the small disk surrounded by a rim of sclera. **(REF:** 4, p. 892**)**

533. (C) Gaze-evoked nystagmus may also dampen and change direction with prolonged eccentric gaze. This is called centripetal nystagmus. **(REF:** 54, p. 923**)**

534. (D) The diagnostic criteria for Reye's syndrome include absence of CSF pleocytosis. Tuberculous meningitis produces symptoms of chronic meningitis, elevated intracranial pressure, abnormal CSF with moderately decreased glucose, elevated protein, and pleocytosis and lymphocytic predominance (usually 100-500 cells). Although most patients will have a positive PPD, it is not imperative. **(REF:** 32, pp. 91-97**)**

535. (A) Hypothermia should not produce loss of consciousness until core body temperature falls below 32°C. Ventricular fibrillation may occur at core body temperatures between 27-30°C. The EEG is slow but of normal amplitude. With rapid rewarming, there is generally no permanent neurologic residual deficit. **(REF:** 41, pp. 238-239**)**

536. (B) A diffuse mixed sensorimotor neuropathy and transverse white lines in the nails are signs of lead intoxication. **(REF:** 57, p. 614**)**

537. (B) Large myelinated fibers are those which conduct vibratory sensation. Myelinated fibers of large diameter conduct more rapidly than do unmyelinated and small myelinated fibers, and, therefore, when large fibers are preserved, action potentials and conduction velocity may be normal. **(REF:** 57, p. 686**)**

538. (E) Shingles is caused by Herpes zoster, which is a different virus from H. simplex. Herpes zoster is caused by the same virus as varicella (chicken pox). Shingles commonly involves cranial nerves. **(REF:** 35, pp. 96-98**)**

539. (E) Becker's muscular dystrophy is an x-linked recessive disorder where symptoms usually present by age 10, and rarely after age 25. Initial weakness is in pelvic and shoulder girdle muscle with spread to limb muscles. Serum CPK activity is moderately elevated and cardiac involvement is quite uncommon. **(REF:** 4, p. 385**)**

540. (C) The question describes the pseudobulbar syndrome. Wallenberg: ipsilateral Horner's, ataxia, facial sensation, palatal elevation and contralateral hemibody spinothalamic dysfunction (lateral medulla). Weber: ipsilateral third nerve paresis and contralateral arm and leg paresis (paramedian mesencephalon). Millard- Gubler: ipsilateral sixth and seventh nerve dysfunction and contralateral arm and leg weakness (paramedian pons). Benedikts: Weber (+) contralateral hemianesthesia and choreiform movements (paramedian mesencepholon). **(REF:** 35, p. 167**)**

541. (C) See Question 540. This is the Weber syndrome.

542. (D) No characteristic symptoms are available which will help differentiate an acute subdural hematoma from cerebral contusion. Both are characterized by headache, fluctuating mental status, focal neurologic deficit (referable) to the locus of brain injury. Symptoms develop within the first few days following head trauma. **(REF:** 35, p. 286**)**

543. (C) Cataplexy is an abrupt reversible loss of postural tone with maintenance of consciousness, often precipitated by strong emotions. It is associated with narcolepsy and is believed to be a dissociated manifestation of REM sleep. It is not a seizure disorder and is not associated with the Kleine-Levin syndrome. **(REF:** 35, p. 659**)**

544. (C) The pattern of deficit does not suggest optic neuritis or multiple sclerosis. The history suggests a syndrome of hereditary optic neuropathy. Although clinically compatible with Leber's disease, Leber's optic atrophy is usually a disease of young men, felt to be transmitted from mother to son. **(REF:** 10, p. 164**)**

545. (C) Although vascular occlusion and ischemic damage to the nervous system may occur in all disease processes listed, giant cell arteritis is the disease entity classically associated with central retinal artery occlusion. This may occur in one-third of cases, resulting in blindness. **(REF:** 10, p. 40**)**

546. (B) Although hypertension, atherosclerosis, diabetes, syphilis, and collagen disease are all associated with the occurrence of cerebrovascular accident, arteriosclerosis is the most common cause of stroke. Atherothrombosis is associated with 70% of strokes. **(REF:** 35, p. 147**)**

547. (C) Leprosy is a disease caused by infection with M. lepral, which produces cutaneous and nervous lesions. An early manifestation is an erythematous nodule, the lepride. Any peripheral nerve may be affected, but there is a predilection for the ulnar, greater auricular, anterior tibial, and cranial nerves V and VII. **(REF:** 35, pp. 63-64**)**

548. (C) Huntington's chorea may present with dementia or personality changes. The average duration of disease is said to be about 15 years. Seizures may be seen frequently in the juvenile variant. Huntington's chorea is transmitted as an autosomal dominant, and both sexes are affected equally. **(REF:** 26, p. 301**)**

549. (E) Acutely following spinal cord transection, spinal shock may occur, producing a temporary paralysis of bladder and bowel function and loss of deep and cutaneous reflexes. **(REF:** 35, p. 300**)**

550. (B) Seizures generally occur 6-18 months following brain injury, occurring in 2-40% of patients. Seizures may be of any type except petit mal and are most often generalized. **(REF:** 35, p. 295**)**

551. (D) The clinical feature cf Friedreich's ataxia include ataxia, sensory loss, nystagmus, depressed DTRs, kyphoscoliosis, optic atrophy, cranial nerve palsies, and mental deterioration. The onset is usually in the first or second decade. **(REF:** 35, p. 500**)**

552. (E) Sensory loss is not characteristic of Shy-Drager syndrome. Pathologically, lesions are found in the cerebellar, pyramidal, extrapyramidal, and autonomic nervous systems. **(REF:** 26, p. 307**)**

553. (C) Wohlfhart-Kugelberg-Welander is a syndrome characterized by progressive proximal neurogenic muscular atrophy. It is distinguished from muscular dystrophies and myositis by EMG and biopsy findings, and from ALS by its slow progression and lack of corticospinal signs. **(REF:** 35, p. 545**)**

554. (B) Physical exam in all of these diseases may indicate upper motor neuron dysfunction referable to the spinal cord. Syringomyelia, however, is most likely to be differential clinically, because of the likelihood of a motor and sensory spinal cord level, and the presence of dissociated sensory loss at the level of the lesion. **(REF:** 35, pp. 553-555**)**

555. (B) The most common location of the syringomyelia cavity is in the lower cervical region. **(REF:** 35, p. 530**)**

556. (C) Of the choices, the classic clinical symptoms are the most reliable means of making the diagnosis of syringomyelia. **(REF:** 35, p. 554**)**

557. (A) Nearly all brains of patients with Down's syndrome contain typical Alzheimer changes. An increase in the number of cases of Down's syndrome among relatives of probands with Alzheimer's disease has been documented. Autoimmune diseases such as thyroid disease are associated with Down's syndrome. **(REF:** 3, pp. 144-145**)**

558. (B) D-penicillamine, polymyxins, and aminoglycosides
559. (C) are among the drugs which can lead to neuromus-
560. (B) cular blockade and a syndrome which resembles the signs and symptoms of myasthenia gravis. Similarly, underlying myasthenia gravis may be aggravated by these agents. Nonsteroidal anti-inflammatory agents do not have this effect. Treatment with neostigmine is often effective during the symptomatic phase of drug-induced myasthenia. High-dose corticosteroids may acutely intensify neuromuscular weakness in this setting. **(REF:** 5, pp. 409-413**)**

561. (A) Ophthalmoplegic migraine occurs mostly in children, equally in boys and girls. The headaches usually occur on the same side as the ophthalmoplegia and may last several days. Visual prodromes are rare. **(REF:** 54, p. 989**)**

562. (B) Adie's or tonic pupil is usually but not exclusively unilateral. It shows degeneration supersensitivity and constricts to dilute pharmacologic solutions. It is often associated with diminished deep tendon reflexes. Pathologically, there have been reported marked loss of memory in the ciliary ganglion, producing postganglionic parasympathetic denervation. **(REF:** 54, p. 867**)**

563. (E) All of these can cause blurring of optic disc margins in the absence of increased intracranial pressure, or "pseudopapilledema." **(REF:** 54, pp. 883-885**)**

564. (C) Rarely SVP are observed with papilledema, when intracranial pressure is normal. Visual acuity is normal in acute papilledema. One cause of increased intracranial pressure, pseudotumor cerebri, may be familial. **(REF:** 54, p. 887**)**

565. (C) Thrombocytopenia, hypofibrinogenemia, and an elevated protime is seen in disseminated intravascular coagulation. Steroids are not indicated in this setting. The neurologic complications include subarachnoid hemorrhage, small and large vessel occlusions, microhemorrhages, embolication from nonbacterial thrombotic endocarditis. **(REF:** 51, pp. 791-797**)**

566. (A) The first three statements are true. Hyperacusis develops as the result of paralysis of the stapedius muscle. The nerve supply to this region originates proximal to the chorda tympani. **(REF:** 15, pp. 1-98**)**

567. (C) Sarcoid involves the nervous system in approximately 5% of patients with sarcoid. It generally produces a low CSF glucose and pleocytosis with lymphocytic predominance. **(REF:** 14, pp. 336-345**)**

568. (A) Epidemiologic study reveals that fibromuscular dysplasia, polycystic kidney, and coarctation of the aorta are all associated with an increased incidence of intracranial aneurysms. Although hypertension may make aneurysm rupture more likely, this is not a proven risk factor for intracranial aneurysm formation. **(REF:** 61, entire chapter**)**

569. (D) The risk of rebleeding is greatest 10 days after the rupture of an intracranial aneurysm, probably due to breakdown of the thrombus which forms initially. This risk stabilizes about 30 days after the event. **(REF:** 61, entire chapter**)**

570. (A) The Vogt-Koyanaji-Harada syndrome is associated with vitiligo, alopecia, meningitis, sensorineural hearing loss, retinal detachments, and papillitis. It is not associated with cardiac conduction abnormalities. **(REF:** 33, entire chapter**)**

571. (A) Lacunar infarcts result from occlusion of small perforating arterial vessels. Valvular disease produces strokes by the mechanism of embolization, affecting large vessels rather than small perforators. **(REF:** 36, pp. 201-222**)**

572. (A) Ataxia hemiparesis syndrome results from lacunar infarcts involving internal capsule or basis pontis, producing weakness of the leg with ipsilateral hemibody incoordination. **(REF:** 36, pp. 201-222**)**

573. (A) Refsum's disease may be controlled by consuming a diet low in phytanic acid. **(REF:** 43, pp. 605-666**)**

574. (B) Fibromuscular dysplasia is characterized by hyperplastic segmental changes in the intima and media of large arteries, most commonly the internal carotid arteries. It is more common in women than men. No intervention is warranted unless symptoms develop. **(REF:** 11, pp. 616-618**)**

575. (D) Drugs which stimulate the synthesis of S-ALA must be avoided. Paraldehyde is the only drug listed which may be used with relative safety in this setting. **(REF:** 44, pp. 480-484**)**

576. (A) Bilateral forebrain dysfunction is associated with
577. (D) posthyperventilation apnea and with Cheyne-
578. (C) Stokes respirations. Pontine disease is associated
579. (A) with apneustic and cluster breathing. Medullary
580. (C) lesions are associated with ataxic breathing. **(REF:** 41, p. 34**)**

581. (D) Leptospirosis, Lyme disease, and syphilis are all
582. (A) caused by spirochetes. Myositis and nephrosis are
583. (B) associated specifically with Leptospiresis. Cryo-
584. (E) globulins are associated with Lyme disease. **(REF:** 52, pp. 172-181**)**

585. (B) Drusen are translucent bodies of the optic nerve head. **(REF:** A, p. 651**)**

586. (A) Devic's disease is a variant of multiple sclerosis characterized by bilateral optic neuritis and transverse myelitis. **(REF:** 10, p. 150**)**

587. (D) Bechet's disease is characterized by recurrent painful orogenital ulcers, ureitis, cranial nerve palsies, seizures, strokes, meningoencephalitis, joint effusions, and thrombophlebitis. **(REF:** 10, p. 150**)**

588. (C) Beri-beri optic neuritis occurs in the setting of dietary deficiency (probably due to vitamin B deficiency) as may occur in P.O.W. camps. **(REF:** 10, p. 150**)**

589. (B) Cerebellar astrocytoma of childhood is a relatively benign, well-circumscribed lesion, which may arise in the hemisphere or vermis. **(REF:** 60, p. 1419**)**

590. (A) The polar spongioblastoma is a rare primitive neuroglial tumor which usually arises in the brainstem adjacent to the third or fourth ventricles. **(REF:** 60, p. 1419**)**

591. (E) The hemangioblastoma occurs most commonly in the fourth decade, accounting for more than 7% of posterior fossa tumors in that age group. **(REF:** 60, p. 1419**)**

592. (D) Medulloblastomas most commonly arise in the cerebellar midline. **(REF:** 60, p. 1419**)**

593. (C) The ependymoma arises from ependymal cells and is typically an intraventricular tumor. The fourth ventricle is the most common intracranial site. **(REF:** 60, p. 1419**)**

594. (C) In both botulism and myasthenia gravis neuromus-
595. (C) cular transmission is abnormal, producing muscle
596. (B) weakness. Botulinum toxia acts as the presynap-
597. (A) tic membrane to interfere with acetylcholine release. Repetitive stimulation produces a successive

increase in end plate potential size (facilitation) in botulism. In myasthenia gravis, repetitive stimulation produces successive decrement in action potential size. **(REF:** 59, pp. 334-353**)**

598. (C) The pattern of chorodial blood vessels and background retinal pigment produces the "tigroid fundus," a normal variant. **(REF:** 64, pp. 365-366**)**

599. (A) Retinitis pigmentosa, characterized by peripheral retinal pigmentary clumps and vascular attenuation. **(REF:** 64, p. 629**)**

600. (D) Hypertensive retinopathy, arteriovenous nicking, and scattered flame-shaped hemorrhages are apparent. **(REF:** 64, pp. 882-888**)**

REFERENCES

1. Adams, R. D. and Sidman, R. *Introduction to Neuropathology.* Blakiston-McGraw Hill, N.Y., 1968.

2. Albers, R. W., Siegel, G. J., Katzman, R., and Agrenoff, B. *Basic Neurochemistry.* Little, Brown and Co., Boston, 1972.

3. Appel, S. M. *Current Neurology,* Vol. 3. John Wiley and Sons, N.Y., 1981.

4. Armbrustmacher, V. W. and Griffin, J. L. "Neuromuscular Diseases" in *The Clinical Neurosciences.* Roger N. Rosenberg (Ed.) Vol. I. Churchill-Livingstone, N.Y., 1983.

5. Argov, Z. and Mastaglia, F. L. "Disorders of neuromuscular transmission caused by drugs." *N. Engl. J. Med.* 409-413, August 23, 1979.

6. Brock, S. and Krieger, H. *The Basis of Clinical Neurology,* 4th Ed. Williams and Wilkins, Baltimore, 1963.

7. Browne, T. R. "Valproic acid," *N. Engl. J. Med.* 661-666 March 20, 1980.

8. Buonamo, F. S. "Neuroimaging" in *Neurologic Clinics,* Vol. 2, #4, November 1984, W. B. Saunders Co., Philadelphia.

9. Chiappa, K. H. and Popper, A. H. "Evoked potentials in clinical medicine." *N Engl. J. Med.* May 13, 1982 and May 20, 1982.

10. Cogen, O. G. *Neurology of the Visual System.* C. Thomas, Springfield, Ill., 1966.

11. Corrin, S., et al. "Cerebral ischemic events in patients with carotid artery fibromuscular dysplosia." *Arch. Neurol.* 38:616-618, October, 1981.

12. Crosby, E., Humphrey, T., and Laver, E. *Correlative Anatomy of the Nervous System.* Macmillan, N.Y., 1962.

13. DeJong, R. *The Neurologic Examination,* 4th Ed. Harper and Row, N.Y., 1979.

14. Delaney, P. "Neurologic manifestations in sarcoidosis." *Ann. Intern. Med.* 87:336-345, 1977.

15. Diamond, C. and Frew, I. *The Facial Nerve.* Oxford University Press, Oxford, 1979.

16. Eccles, J. *The Physiology of Synapses.* Springer-Verlag, Berlin, Connecticut, 1964.

17. Farmer, T. *Pediatric Neurology,* 3rd Ed. Harper and Row, N.Y., 1983.

18. Fuster, V. and Chesebro, J. "Antithrombotic therapy: Role of platelet inhibitor drugs, Part II." *Mayo Clinic Proc.* 56:185-272, March, 1981.

19. Giesser, B. Landry-Guillain-Barré Syndrome." *Resident Staff Physician* 29(8), August, 1983.

20. Goodman, L. and Gilman, A. *The Pharmacological Basis of Therapeutics,* 5th Ed. Macmillan, N.Y., 1975.

21. Gree, R. *Current Concepts of Migraine Research.* Raven Press, N.Y., 1978.

22. Greenfield, J. *Neuropathology,* 3rd Ed. Williams and Wilkins, Baltimore, 1976.

23. Hahn, T. J. "Bone complications of anticonvulsants." *Drugs* 12:201-211, 1976.

24. Haymaker, W. and Woodhall, B. *Peripheral Nerve Injuries,* 2nd Ed. W. B. Saunders, Philadelphia, 1962.

25. Hassler, R. G. and Christ, J. J. (Eds.) *Advances in Neurology,* Vol. 40. Raven Press, N.Y., 1984.

26. Hirano, A. and Llena, J. F. "Degenerative Diseases of the Nervous System" in *The Clinical Neurosciences.* Roger N. Rosenberg (Ed.) Vol. III. Churchill-Livingstone, N.Y., 1983.

27. Junck, L. "Neurotoxicity of radiological contrast agents." *Ann. Neurol.* 13:469-484, 1983.

28. Katz, B. *Nerve, Muscle and Synapse.* McGraw-Hill, N.Y., 1966.

29. Kimura, J. "Principles and pitfalls of nerve conduction studies." *Ann. Neurol.* 16:(4), October 1984.

30. Krigman, M. R. and Bouldin, T. W. "Intoxications and Deficiency Diseases" in *The Clinical Neurosciences,* Vol. 3. Roger Rosenberg (Ed.). Churchill-Livingstone, N.Y., 1983.

31. Kutt, H. and McDowell, F. *Clinical Neuropharmacology.* Churchill-Livingstone, N.Y., 1979.

32. Lehrich, R. R., et al. "Case records of the Mass. Gen. Hospital." *N. Engl. J. Med.* 306:91-97, January 14, 1982.

33. Manor, R. J. "Vogt-Koyanogi- Harada Syndrome and Related Disease" in *Handbook of Clinical Neurology.* Vinken, P. J. and Bruyn, G. W. (Eds.) Vol. 34. North Holland, Amsterdam, 1978.

34. Merritt, J. L. "Management of spasticity." *Mayo Clinic Proc.* 56:614, 1981.

35. Merritt, H. *A Textbook of Neurology,* 7th Ed. Lea and Febiger, Philadelphia, 1984.

36. Mohr, J. P. *Lacunes, Neurologic Clinics,* Vol. 1, No. 1. W. B. Saunders Co., Philadelphia, February 1983.

37. Mountcastle, V. *Medical Physiology.* Mosby, St. Louis, MO, 1968.

38. Onfrig, M., et al. "Dopaminergic deficiency causes delayed VEPs in rats." *Ann. Neurol.* 11:484-490, 1982.

39. Parke, S. W., Richardson, E. O. and McCormick, G. F. "Case records of the Mass. Gen. Hosp." *N. Engl. J. Med.* 1925-1931, November 29, 1984.

40. Penry, J. K. and Newmark, M. E. "The use of antiepileptic drugs." *Ann. Intern. Med.* 90:207-218, 1979.

41. Plum, F. and Posner, J. *The Diagnosis of Stupor and Coma,* 3rd Ed. F. A. Davis Co., Philadelphia, 1980.

42. Powers, J. M. *"Metabolic Diseases of the Nervous System"* in The Clinical Neurosciences. Roger Rosenberg (Ed.) Vol. III. Churchill-Livingstone, Boston, 1983.

43. Refsum, S. "Heredopathica atactica polyneuritiformis." *Arch. Neurol.* 31:605-666, October 1981.

44. Reynolds, N. C. and Miska, R. M. "Safety of Anticonvulsants in hepatic porphyria." *Neurology* 31:480-484, April 1984.

45. Rodriquez, M., Powell, H. C., and Lampert, P. "Demyelination and Leukodystrophy" in *The Clinical Neurosciences.* Roger N. Rosenberg (Ed.) Vol. III. Churchill-Livingstone, N.Y., 1983.

46. Rose, J. Q., et al. "Intoxication caused by interaction of chloramphenicol and phenytoin." *JAMA* 237(24), 1977.

47. Rubinstein, L. J. *Tumors of the Central Nervous System.* Armed Forces Institute of Pathology, Washington, D.C., 1972.

48. Ruch, T. and Patton, H. *Physiology and Biophysics.* 20th Ed. W. B. Saunders, Philadelphia, 1979, Vol. I and 1982, Vol. IV.

49. Samuels, M. A. (Ed.) *Manual of Neurologic Therapeutics,* 2nd Ed. Little, Brown Co., Boston, p. 309, 1982.

50. Schaumburg, H. H., Spencer, P. S., and Thomas, P. K. *Disorders of Peripheral Nerves.* F. A. Davis Co., Philadelphia, 1983.

51. Schwartzman, R. J. and Hill, J. B. "Neurologic complications of disseminated intravascular coagulation." *Neurology,* 32:791-797, August, 1982.

52. Scully, R. E., et al. "Case records of the Mass. Gen. Hospital." *N. Engl. J. Med.* 311:(3), July 19, 1984, pp. 172-181.

53. Siegel, G. J., Albers, R. W., Agranoff, B., and Katzman, R. *Basic Neurochemistry,* 3rd Ed. Little, Brown and Co., Boston, 1983.

54. Smith, C. H. and Beck, R. W. *Neurophthalmology,* Neurologic Clinics, Vol. 1, No. 4. W. B. Saunders Co., Philadelphia, November 1983.

55. Spark, R. F. and Dickstein, G. "Bromocriptine and endocrine disorders." *Ann. Intern. Med.* 90:949-956, 1979.

56. Spehlman, R. *EEG Primer.* Elsevier North Holland, Amsterdam, 1981.

57. Spencer, P. S. and Schaumburg, H. H. (Eds.) *Experimental and Clinical Neurotoxicology.* Williams and Wilkins, Baltimore, 1980.

58. Stockard, J. J., et al. *Mayo Clinic Proc.* 52:761-769, 1977.

59. Swift, T. R. "Disorders of neuromuscular transmission other than myasthenia gravis." *Muscle and Nerve* 4:334-353, July-August 1981.

60. Taveras, J. and Wood, E. *Diagnostic Neuroradiology.* Williams and Wilkins, Baltimore, 2nd Ed. 1976.

61. Tew, J. M. "Guidelines for Management and Surgical Treatment of Intracranial Aneurysms" in *Controversies in Neurology.* Thompson, R. A. and Green, J. R. (Eds.) Raven Press, N.Y., 1983.

62. Truex, R. and Carpenter M. *Human Neuroanatomy,* 6th Ed. Williams and Wilkins, Baltimore, 1969.

63. Wagner, D. R. and Weitzman, E. D. "Sleep and Arousal Disorders" in *The Clinical Neurosciences.* Roger N. Rosenberg (Ed.) Vol. 1:879, Churchill-Livingstone, N.Y., 1983.

64. Walsh, F. B. *Clinical Neurophthalmology,* 2nd Ed. Williams and Wilkins, Baltimore, 1957.

65. Zemon, V., et al. "Bicuculline enhances a negative component and diminishes a positive component of the VEP in the cat." *Proc. Nat. Acad. Sci., USA* 77:7976-7978, 1980.

A. Ballantyne, A. J. and Michaelson, I. C. *Textbook of the Fundus of the Eye,* Williams and Wilkins, Baltimore, 1970.

B. Guze, B. H. and Baxter, L. R. "Current concepts: Neuroleptic malignant syndrome." *N. Engl. J. Med.* 313(3):163-165, July 18, 1985.